AIN'T DEAD YET

Winning a Wrestling Match Against Guillain-Barré

Danny Freeman

Mountain Page Press

HENDERSONVILLE, NC

M

Published 2020, 2021 by Mountain Page Press

ISBN 978-1-952714-27-6

Second Edition
Copyright © 2020 Danny Freeman

First Edition
Copyright © 2019 Danny Freeman

For information, contact the publisher at:
Mountain Page Press
118 5th Ave. W.
Hendersonville, NC 28792

Visit: www.MountainPagePress.com

This is a work of creative non-fi ction. All of the events in this memoir are true to the best of the author's memory. Some names and identifying features have been changed to protect the identity of certain parties.

The views expressed in this memoir are solely those of the author.

Dedication

I dedicate my story to those of you who
have suffered with Guillain-Barré Syndrome,
and to your families and friends.

This is also dedicated to those who experience any
debilitating event in life. May you find the
strength that I found to persevere.

CONTENTS

PROLOGUE

The one thing that is certain about life is that everything is uncertain. There's no way that we can know what will take place next week, tomorrow, in the next hour, or in the next minute—or second, for that matter. You may have a good idea of what will happen, and you may often be correct in your prediction—but it's still not a certainty. It's just a prediction.

If we all knew beyond a shadow of a doubt what would take place in the future, civilization would cease to exist. Uncertainty is what drives the economy. It's what drives our everyday existence and development. If we all knew what was coming up next, then everyone would either be incredibly wealthy—or destitute. There must be contrast, and uncertainty is what creates this contrast.

I've been somewhat of a gambler all my life, but any truthful gambler will tell you an important fact. If you gamble long enough, even though you may have been on a hot streak, sooner or later it will even out. If not, gaming meccas such as Las Vegas, Atlantic City, and Monte Carlo would all collapse; and the last time I checked, they were all expanding by leaps and bounds.

Most religions speak of prophets who can predict the future through faith. I've never understood the claim that you hear of these correct prophecies in the past tense. It's always,

"He or she prophesized three or four years ago that this or that would take place." Why did no one hear of these predictions three or four years ago and carry out steps to guard against or to profit from the prediction?

When it all comes down to it, no one can predict the future. We're at the mercy of destiny, and there's not a thing we can do about it. We can try to influence what will transpire, but there's no guarantee.

What we can control, however, is how we react to these changes coming at us constantly from all sides. Most of the changes are small. Some are even so minute they're acted upon by instinct. They require no conscious thought; we just deal with them as they come—without even considering what would have happened had our reactions been different. That's the way day-to-day life operates. Nothing can be done about these occurrences. We handle them automatically.

What I'll attempt to convey in this book is how I've dealt with changes and experiences during my life. I'm now sixty years old, and I've been told by most people who are privy to my life story that I have lived—as they put it—a full life. I feel that a lot can be learned from things I've been through and how I reacted to them—and I will try to make it a bit entertaining along the way.

The main theme of my story is to stay as positive in your mindset as possible when you encounter adversity. When you face a serious situation, this is often difficult to accomplish. These situations can run the gamut from affairs of the heart, to the death of a loved one, to monetary disasters, or anything else that may adversely affect your life.

My story touches on several of these events in one way or another, but the core of my book is dedicated to a medical issue that slammed me up against a wall and nearly killed me.

Life-changing events can alter one's existence in the blink of an eye and can result in either a negative ending, or—as I will try to get across here—in a positive one. Hopefully I provide a way to assist others when they are blindsided by extreme adversity. I've learned a lot along the way. I didn't make all the right decisions, but I did make some—or I wouldn't be here writing this today.

I believe that the greatest teacher is history. We can acquire a tremendous amount of practical knowledge by looking at how others have confronted similar situations. I would much rather learn from someone who has actually been through an experience than from someone who never went.

In this case, I get to honestly tell you that I've actually been there—and made it back to tell of the trip. I hope you enjoy my story.

CHAPTER ONE

FIRST SIX WEEKS

September 24, 2015 started as most of my days did back then.

I got up, had my morning constitutional, and took a shower. I always took a shower in the same order. First, I washed my face, then my upper body, paying particular attention to my underarms, then my private parts, legs, and feet. I often wondered if other people took a shower in the same way. Probably so, but that's just not something you bring up in daily conversation. I then brushed my teeth and shaved. This would be the last day I would do these things for myself for six months.

I dressed in business casual attire as I most often did, in polo shirts and khaki pants; then I went to prison. I should specify here that I went to work in a prison. I was in my twentieth year with the North Carolina Department of Correction. Little did I know that this would also be my last day of work.

I walked through the gatehouse, security, and finally through the doors to the lobby, the sally port (a series of security gates) at master control, and then down the elevated hallway to the F-Unit housing area, for which I was responsible.

The hallway was elevated because the prison was built on a huge rock formation, and the cost of leveling the steep incline at that spot would have been too great, so the contractors just built over the top of it. Over the years, it became known as "The Rock." An apt name for a maximum security prison, I thought.

Back on May 6, 1996, I started at the bottom as a Correctional Officer at Marion Correctional Institution, just a year after it opened. I've seen a lot of unusual things in my life—which you'll learn about—but that first day was truly frightening. It was nothing like what I'd seen in the movies or on TV.

I was still in my orientation phase when a lieutenant took us on a tour of the custody section, the area where the inmates lived. Murderers, rapists, thieves, molesters, and the like—all living in cells. Each cell had a heavy metal door that could be opened only by hitting a switch in a central control room or overriding the switch with a key. The inmates we saw that day were pretty much all out in the dayroom, which was a central location in each housing wing. This was disturbing to me as I had always envisioned prisoners behind bars. Bars were used, but only to prevent access to larger parts of the institution. The tour continued, and I walked along thinking, "What have I gotten myself into?"

The city of Marion is the county seat of McDowell County, nestled in the foothills of the majestic Blue Ridge Mountains in Western North Carolina. I was born and raised there, though my travels and adventures frequently took me far away from my hometown. Marion Correctional is a huge institution that houses minimum and maximum security prisoners—one of only three of that size in the state at the time. It was designated as maximum security, or as the state of North Carolina calls it, close custody, with a capacity of 720 inmates. I began my career there after owning and operating a full line pet store, an occupation that started out to be extremely profitable until we saw the opening of a store called Walmart. You may have heard of it. I'd been competing with them for seven years, and by this time I was still paying the bills, but barely.

I had a couple of long-time friends who had worked at our local minimum security facility for several years, so I contacted them for advice. I couldn't see myself being a correctional officer for long, so I asked about my options in regard to promotional possibilities if I was hired. They both told me that the opportunities were excellent, as the institution employed over 400 people; and between attrition and in-house promotions, jobs would regularly open up through the chain of command. So I applied, interviewed, and was hired. I had a going-out-of-business sale at the pet store, and I was off to start a new career, which would turn out to be the lengthiest of my life.

I moved up through the ranks at the prison pretty quickly. I spent two years as an officer, (the minimum time for promotion in the custody section), then four years as a sergeant, and then the next fourteen years in unit management. Unit managers and assistant unit managers are responsible for overseeing the operation of one of the prison's four housing units. Each unit housed a maximum of 192 inmates. Maximum capacity was the norm. The authority level of a unit manager was equivalent to that of a captain in this paramilitary environment. The job became extremely stressful at that point, and I didn't know if I wanted to do it anymore.

I decided to make a change, and in June 2015 I transitioned into a newly created position as a Career Readiness Coach. This primarily involved the recruitment of new, frontline officers and nurturing them through their first two years of employment in an attempt to reduce turnover. The goal was, as the job title implies, to assist new officers to make corrections a career as I had done. This turned out to be more than a job for me. I loved it. My years as an instructor for the department, coupled with my natural desire to help new staff members adapt to an alien atmosphere, was very rewarding. With that, the desire to excel in my new profession returned. As it turned out, this would be a short-lived opportunity.

Thursday, September 24, 2015
7:30 A.M.
Clad in my khakis and a polo shirt, I made my fifteen minute drive to work as I did every day. I took the back roads to get there, as was my habit. This relaxed me in anticipation of working in a stressful environment. I spent a normal day on the job, just like every other day.

5:00 P.M.
I made the short drive after work out to the local YMCA and went through my usual: a 45 to 60 minute workout, which always felt great. No problem. I wiped off the sweat, drove home, and proceeded to spend an evening at home.

I should point out here that I have never been married. I came close a couple of times, but it never came to fruition for various reasons. As a result, I live in the home where I grew up in the small community of Nebo, North Carolina; the one I had purchased when my father passed away in 2003. My mother died in 1997, less than a year after I had started my career with the prison system.

8:00 P.M.

I enjoyed the company of a young lady from time to time in this home, but on this particular evening I was by myself. Everything was completely normal. I sat down, relaxed, watched TV in the den (which I had turned into my man cave), and ate a dinner that I had prepared myself. I rarely ate fast food because my previous travels had made me appreciate a home-cooked meal more than anything that comes out of a drive-through.

10:00 P.M.

I decided to pack it in for the night.

11:30 P.M.

I awoke and had to go to the bathroom. The only health problem I had up to this point was an inability to completely empty my bladder, which meant I had to urinate frequently. My doctor called it an "inability to void." I had been checked out for this, but no solution was determined. More tests had been scheduled soon.

Anyway, I got up and noticed a numbness on my right side. I wrote it off because I was a side-sleeper for the most part and assumed I had just slept wrong. I used the bathroom, turned around, and started walking back to my bed—and stumbled. It felt as if my knees had buckled. I reached out with my hands and caught myself between the bathroom counter and wall to keep myself from falling. I tentatively made my way back to my bed and wrote it off as getting my feet tangled up, as I didn't wear my contacts while I slept and had extremely poor vision without them.

11:30 P.M.

I lay back down and quickly felt the numbness spreading down my left side. I became concerned. Within a matter of a few minutes, the numbness grew across my mid-section. By this time, I knew something was wrong. I decided to get up on my feet and confirm that the incident in the bathroom was just a freak occurrence. I turned around, sat up on the edge of the bed, and attempted to stand up. I only proved that the incident in the bathroom wasn't random—I nearly fell into the dresser. Something was seriously wrong. I thought perhaps I was having a stroke. I had my cell phone on the nightstand as always, so I called 911. Luckily, the Emergency Medical Services (EMS) had established a local substation only about a mile from my home a couple of years before. This station had been funded, along with a huge fire department, by the many residents who occupied the nearby lakeside developments.

The story of how the lake had been developed is interesting. My best friend, a fellow by the name of Bracey Bobbitt, had made a deal with Crescent Timber, which was the land-holding entity of our statewide power company, Duke Energy, which had created Lake James as a power-producing source back in 1917. Crescent Timber decided to sell the land around the lake that wasn't privately owned, and Bracey was the first one to purchase parcels.

Bracey's first developments were adjacent to our only local golf course, The Marion Lake Club. He bought several plots of land and developed them into small, extremely nice homes, along with parcels of land left as building sites.

He created three housing developments, one of which was called North Shores. In fact, he asked me to serve as secretary for the corporation when his ex-wife was no longer able to fill the position. In order to form a corporation, only three positions had to be established: president, vice president, and secretary. One person was allowed to occupy up to two positions. Bracey served as both president and vice president. The duty of secretary entailed nothing more than going to a local attorney's office when a sale was made, signing the paperwork, and establishing a seal on said paperwork. For that I received $100 for my time. So, the development of homes on the lake down from my house necessitated the building of emergency services nearby. At any rate, that's the reason the EMS substation was located so near to me. You never know when this'll come in handy, huh?

11:40 P.M.

The EMS personnel arrived in about five minutes, and I was happy to see that one of the two people on duty was a fellow named Donnie, whom I had known for many years. He came in and we discussed my symptoms, and he and the other Emergency Medical Technician assisting him agreed that I may have been experiencing a stroke. They had to help me toward the gurney, which they had left in my kitchen. I managed to make it to the dining room, where I awkwardly sat down in a chair. The gurney was only about ten feet from my position, and without being able to place an arm around each of their shoulders, I couldn't have made it on my own. That was how quickly my strength deteriorated.

Little did I know that this was as mobile as I was going to be for a very long time.

As they loaded me into the ambulance, my brother Terry came down from his home right behind mine because the ambulance lights woke him up. He asked what was wrong, and I told him that I didn't know for sure, but thought I was having a stroke. I saw him again in the emergency room a few hours later. I normally saw Terry daily, but this was the last time I remembered seeing him for several weeks.

Friday, September 25
12:00 A.M.

I was transported to McDowell Hospital, about fifteen minutes away. There, all the tests one would receive when exhibiting signs of a stroke were conducted, including an EKG. They all came up negative. I was examined by several doctors and nurses on duty that night, but no one could come up with an explanation for my rapid loss of strength and my still deteriorating condition.

I remained in the emergency room the rest of that night, shuffled from one small area to another as new patients came in with various ailments that required urgent care. I was sequestered to a chair in a small room at the back of the ER where, as it turned out, I was to remain overnight with no diagnosis and little attention.

6:00 A.M.

As morning approached, I telephoned one of my oldest friends, Duane Terrell, who had worked his way up to super-intendent of the prison. Duane had since retired, but he and I had remained close friends, as we had been since childhood. He and his wife, Debbie, would turn out to be crucial to my well-being during my ordeal—which, unbeknownst to me, had already begun. I told Duane what had happened to me over the previous hours, and he was soon by my side as a much needed friend and advocate.

7:00 A.M.

As morning arrived, so did a shift change. New doctors entered the ER where I remained undiagnosed, feeling ignored. Apparently, my condition was discussed widely, as soon, several physicians came to talk to me. By this time, I was barely able to sit upright in the chair and I was in significant pain.

10:00 A.M.

Sometime during the morning—which turned into afternoon—a doctor and nurse, whose names I regrettably don't remember, told me and the other doctors that I was exhibiting all the symptoms of something called Guillain-Barré (gee-YAH-buh-RAY) Syndrome. They said the only way to determine if this was indeed the case was to perform a spinal tap. The spinal fluid would then be analyzed; and if it displayed an extremely high amount of white blood cells, this would almost certainly confirm the diagnosis.

Guillain-Barré is an illness which, for unknown reasons, causes the immune system to attack the nervous system, destroying the myelin sheath, which acts as an insulator that surrounds every nerve in the body. When a nerve is exposed, it causes brain signals sent to the muscles to—for lack of a better term—short out. This hinders the muscle from being able to perform its normal function and it stops working.

This illness affects only about 1 in every 100,000 people worldwide each year, and I had never heard of it.

Considering my failing condition and my hope-filled faith in doctors, I agreed to the spinal tap. The only problem was that McDowell, a relatively small hospital, had no fluoroscope, the machine needed to view inside the body to determine exactly where to insert the needle for the procedure. I'd have to rely solely on the skill of the doctor performing the procedure to get it right.

The doctor performing the procedure wasn't the same as the one who had diagnosed it, but I still had confidence in him. He seemed to know what he was doing, and was also genuinely concerned. For the procedure, I had to lie on a table and turn onto my right side. This proved to be quite a chore, as I had lost about 70 percent of my strength. It was accomplished by the staff with a little help from me, and I was finally in position for the exacting procedure—one that could determine my destiny.

The doctor selected a point along the lower portion of my spine and inserted a rather large needle. I know the word *needle* may make you cringe; but I have no fear of needles. In fact, back in the late '80s, I made my living as a professional wrestler; and at that time I regularly used steroids, which I sometimes I injected myself. In that business, the better you looked, the more money and attention you received.

The first attempt into my spine produced no fluid, and thus, no success. I was asked if it would be alright to make a second attempt in a different spot. I agreed to it.

The second attempt was made just a little higher on my spine—again with no result. Let me make it clear, you do not want this to be performed on you in any condition, even with a local anesthetic. It was extremely painful—and fruitless.

3:00 P.M.

Making no headway, doctors decided to transfer me to the nearest high tech hospital, Mission Health Care in Asheville, North Carolina, about thirty-five minutes away. I was taken by ambulance with no lights or sirens; those things weren't needed because I wasn't in critical condition—yet.

4:00 P.M.

The first thing they did at Mission was to place me face-down on some type of examining table. They then used a fluoroscope and pinpointed where they needed to explore the inner reaches of my spine. I was given another local anesthetic and the doctor inserted the needle, which wasn't painful at all. The spinal fluid he withdrew revealed an extraordinarily high number of white blood cells. I was immediately taken into the Intensive Care Unit (ICU). A short time later, another doctor came in and explained that I had indeed contracted Guillain-Barré Syndrome. He also explained the details of the illness. I listened intently and put my care utterly in his hands. I had no reason not to.

The situation progressed, and in under twenty-four hours of my first symptoms, I found myself almost completely paralyzed. As is true with most people who suffer this horrific disease, I could still move my head and speak, as well as shrug my shoulders. All other muscular functions in my body had shut down. This was a bit unsettling, but the only thing in my mind at the time was, *I'm in a top-notch hospital and they will fix me.*

The only other times I had been in a hospital up to this point were when I had a tonsillectomy at age three, and shoulder replacement and hip replacement surgeries eight and five years previous, respectively. The later two procedures were both predetermined by gradually increasing pain, necessitating the need for each. The shoulder replacement undoubtedly came from years of playing baseball growing up, and the hip issue probably came from both normal wear and tear and my short-lived wrestling career. I spent minimal time in a hospital for each procedure and had no fear or doubt that whatever was happening to me this time would be quickly solved.

I was mistaken.

Many times since then, I've been asked if I was scared. I can honestly say I wasn't. I had confidence in the staff and in the fact that I had kept myself in good physical condition up to that day. I would later discover that if I had not been in good physical shape going into my illness, the coming days would likely have killed me.

The next few days involved attempts to stabilize my condition. Since I was in the ICU, there was a limit on how many visitors I could have and how long they could stay. Many of my closest friends showed up those first few days, and I talked easily with them. It wouldn't be long before this was not the case.

The doctors told me that the first step in stabilizing me was the administration of an intravenous solution called Immune Globulin (IGIV). The IGIV was to be administered for five days, by which time I should be on the road to recovery. I also remember one of the doctors telling me that the cost of the treatment was incredibly expensive. I took this into account, but I really didn't care, as it looked as if I was in for a lengthy hospital stay anyway. I would depend on my Blue Cross insurance, which I received from the state as a benefit for working for the Department of Public Safety (a term

serving as a moniker for several divisions such as prisons—
the largest—the Highway Patrol, etc.). At any rate, cost meant
nothing to me.

September 26

The IV solution took a day to arrive and was administered immediately. I vividly remember looking up at the IGIV
bag hanging beside the regular IV bag, which delivered, I
imagine, a saline solution to keep me hydrated. It struck me
that the IGIV bag was less than half the size of the saline bag.
I remember thinking, This must be some powerful stuff if
such a small amount of medicine can get me back to normal.

For the next five days, my routine consisted of watching
TV and looking up at that bag about every thirty minutes to
make sure it was getting smaller, knowing it was dripping
some substance into my body to cure me. During this time
a feeding tube was inserted into my stomach, just below the
left side of my rib cage—so now my meals also came out of
a bag. I remember the food in the bag was light brown, but I
had no idea what it contained. I loved eating a good meal as
much as anyone, and over the years of living mostly alone, I
had become quite the chef.

During the next several months, I'd realize just how much
being able to eat solid food meant to me. It's one of those
things we take for granted that's actually extremely important to us. There's a sense of anticipation while you prepare
the food, smell it cooking, and dress it to taste just the way
you want. We're also accustomed to the mouth feel of different flavors, textures, and temperatures. I can't relate to you
just how much—as time wore on—I wanted a good, sloppy,
greasy, cheeseburger.

September 30

At the end of the five days, the IGIV treatment had not produced the results desired; and they extended my treatment two more days. *No problem,* I thought. *Just forty-eight hours and I'll start getting back to normal.* You'd be right to guess that this did not happen.

October 1

At the end of that seven days, a doctor—whose name I again regret not remembering—stood at my bed and delivered the sobering news. Since the IGIV hadn't worked, the only alternative was to begin a series of plasma exchanges that might stop the progression of the disease. Again, I thought, *No problem, there will be another treatment if that doesn't work.*

Then the doctor gave me real reason for concern. He told me that since Guillain-Barré was so rare, there had been very little research done on the disease—and therefore, there were few resources for additional treatments. He went on to tell me that, due to the severity of my case, there was a better-than-average chance that my internal organs would begin to shut down. If this happened, they would have to sedate me and start using external support mechanisms. I remember asking him point blank, "Are you going to put me into a coma?" He told me that it wouldn't be an actual comatose state, but I would be strongly sedated. For the first time, I became genuinely concerned.

November 7

I don't remember a lot of the previous six weeks. I do remember waking up occasionally, and there was always a football game on the TV positioned at the foot of my bed. I have no idea if this actually took place—or whether I just imagined it. Hell, sometimes I wasn't sure there even was a TV. During this time, I also experienced a long series of dreams, some more vivid than others. I'll get into the vivid ones later. The ones I encountered at this point weren't that striking. These felt as if I was dreaming in a fog.

I found out later that, during these first six weeks, I came close to death. I was placed on the critical list, and visitors were restricted to immediate family. I have few immediate family members, so I presume I didn't have many visitors at all for quite a while. If I did, I sure don't remember them. I was in a state of limbo between life and death that few people experience.

Let me say at this point that I have never been a religious person. My lack of belief stems from an experience I had as a small child. My older brother was born with a severe case of cerebral palsy. Larry was never able to speak, feed himself, or take care of himself in any way. He required twenty-four-hour care, which my parents provided. Mama and Daddy were both cotton mill workers. Mill work was hard, as I was to discover first-hand many years later. My parents attended a local Baptist church, but after my sister and I were born, they didn't have the time or energy to go anymore, as Sunday was their only day off from work. Cotton mills operated on a six or seven day work schedule, and my parents were wrung out between working and caring for Larry (who was eight years old), three-year-old me, and my baby sister.

After a few missed Sundays, some men from the church, including the preacher, stopped by the house. Mama and Daddy thought this was nice because they assumed the visitors were coming over to check on our welfare and see if the church could help out during a difficult time. What my parents were told changed my mother's life; and even though I didn't know it then, their message changed my life forever too.

My parents were informed that if they were unable to attend services, the church generously offered to send someone by the house to collect the weekly tithe.

You should know that my mama was probably the strongest willed person I have ever known. She had her own beliefs and took no shit from anyone. She was also one of the most caring and compassionate souls I ever knew. But you did not tell her what to do.

The "generous offer" from the church people did not sit well with Mama, and she made that clear to them in no uncertain terms. She also swore that for the rest of her life, she would never set foot in a church again. And she never did.

Even though I was only three years old, I remember this scene vividly. As I look back to what I learned that day and add to it what I have learned over the rest of my life, all these things have fashioned my views regarding religion. I am not an atheist, but I am far from being a devout Christian either. I believe this helped me out during my lengthy time hanging out near death. I wasn't pulling for either team. I was just pulling for myself, and I truly believe that, when the chips are down and it doesn't look good at all, belief in yourself is what it all comes down to.

I've been asked many times what got me through this incredibly difficult experience, and I know what the great majority of people asking the question want my answer to be. Instead, I answer truthfully that I feel what got me through it was trust in myself and in the doctors, nurses, CNAs, and other staff taking care of me. I truly believe this, and I will give no other response. I give credit to the upbringing provided to me by my Mama.

While I'm on this topic, let me tell you a little story about how ol' Danny came to exist in the first place. You see, I almost didn't happen at all. I've already pointed out that my older brother was afflicted with a severe case of cerebral palsy. This was in the 1950s; and in the '50s it was thought that if you had one child with specail needs, you'd better not try to have another one—or it would turn out to be in the same shape or worse than the first one. So, after my brother's birth, my parents resigned themselves to the fact that their dream of having a large family would never come to fruition.

However, in the mid to late '50s, a German doctor by the name of F. J. Ragaz opened a practice in our small town; and for whatever reason, my mother scheduled an appointment with him. Mama would get frustrated with doctors and dentists at the drop of a hat if they didn't tell her what she wanted to hear or if they treated her in a manner that she did not deem appropriate. In other words, if you pissed her off, she had no qualms about going elsewhere. Thank goodness someone pissed her off way back then.

She sat down and talked to Dr. Ragaz, who explained to her that in Europe they didn't hold to the belief that any subsequent births would also result in handicapped offspring. In fact, in Europe it wasn't even considered, and he encouraged my parents to pursue having a family if they so desired. They thought about it and decided to give it a try. This was no small decision back in those days, and I remember Mama telling me many times that a lot of their friends thought they were crazy for making this decision. At any rate, in early 1958 my mother became pregnant with a little boy who would be named Daniel Lee Freeman.

The story of my actual birth is another experience worthy of being told. It was October 6, 1958, at Marion General Hospital in Marion, North Carolina. My mother, a woman named MaeBelle Freeman, was taken into the delivery room, as it appeared she was about to give birth to a baby who was a week overdue. Dr. F. J. Ragaz was the physician in charge. As the labor intensified it became apparent that the baby was going to be born breech—butt first instead of head-first. Giving birth to an 8 lb. 9 oz. baby is normally difficult enough, but when that baby is folded in half, it's much more painful and dangerous to infant and mother. Back in 1958 an epidural or anesthesia of any sort was rare and pretty much nonexistent. C-sections were not performed nearly as often as they are today. As I started to come into the world, Mama kept passing out from the pain, and Dr. Ragaz had to slap her across the face to keep her conscious.

Dr. Ragaz yelled, "Belle, it's my job to keep you alive and to bring this baby into the world; but understand that the baby comes first, and I'm going to do everything in my power to see that it makes it!"

Finally, the nurse told Mama that she had just given birth to an 8 lb. 9 oz. baby boy. Back then there were no ultra-sounds, and you didn't know the sex of your baby until it was born. The nurse told Mama, "I want you to see the first thing your young son did in his life."

My mother looked up at the overhead mirror to see the nurse wiping the little boy's rear end. That's right, sports fans, my first action in my new world was to shit all over myself. A sign of things to come? We'll see.

**

Around the first week of November, my body finally stabilized; and I was moved out of ICU. I vaguely remember a doctor explaining my condition. He touched on the basics of what had happened over the previous six weeks, but didn't go into any detail. I wanted to know more, but I was unable to ask because I had been placed on a ventilator due to my failing lungs. I found out later that many of my internal organs had shut down except for my heart, liver, and kidneys.

Being unable to talk would prove to be one of the most frustrating aspects of my illness. The paralysis had intensified to the point that I could not even use my facial muscles. I couldn't smile. I couldn't frown. And other than my eyelids opening and closing involuntarily, I couldn't move anything anywhere on my body.

I was conscious though! In my mind this was quite an accomplishment. After a day or so, I was moved to Mission's sister facility, St. Joseph's Hospital, across Biltmore Avenue from Mission. St. Joseph's was a much older hospital, which had, at one time, been predominantly staffed by Catholic nuns. I was initially placed in an isolation room because I tested falsely positive on a tuberculosis (TB) test. This was not unusual for me, as I had shown false positive readings from time to time during our annual TB test at the prison.

I remember having a few visitors while I was in isolation. I think my friend Duane was the first one. Duane and his wife Deb were the rocks I leaned on throughout my entire hospitalization.

Every one of my visitors was required to don a surgical gown and a mask and hairnet. I remember lying there, looking up at them standing around my bed in that garb, and not being able to communicate in any way, shape, or form. It was surreal—like something out of a horror movie. At least that's the way it felt through my randomly blinking eyes, which communicated nothing to anyone.

My visitors had a completely different impression; at least that's what I've been told. Through their eyes they were seeing Big Dan in a hell-of-a-lot better shape than he had been over the previous weeks. Being conscious again not only gave me hope and inspiration, it gave hope and inspiration to them as well. Being conscious was a big positive after an extended period of grave, negative news. Visitors proved to be an invaluable inspiration to me.

The visits would increase in frequency during my stay at St. Joseph's, becoming not just an inspiration, but as odd as it may seem, a source of responsibility as well. In my mind I said, *If these people care enough to take the time and effort to visit with someone who can't communicate with them, then I sure can't let them down. I've got to succeed!*

As I look back over my life, my drive to accomplish goals for my benefit, and many times for the benefit of others, is a common theme. The responsibility may have been to live up to my parents' wishes, my friends' wishes, my teammates' wishes, my co-workers' wishes, my employees' wishes . . . the list goes on and on. And that's a good thing. I've achieved many great accomplishments by refusing to let others down. More people should adopt this way of thinking and abandon the mindset of, *It's not worth doing if I don't benefit from it directly.* Benefiting indirectly by living up to the expectations of your fellow man can be even more rewarding, not only for yourself, but for all concerned.

My time at St. Joseph's was pivotal in my recovery. I was moved out of isolation after a couple of days when they determined I wasn't TB contagious. They moved me to room 404 in the Long Term Acute Care unit—the LTAC floor. I was still completely immobile, but cognizant of my situation. My doctor was a guy by the name of Ronnie Jacobs. He was probably fifty years old, a few years younger than me. I turned fifty-seven while in the ICU—a birthday I'll never get back. For some reason this makes me reflect on my old best friend Bracey, who died at fifty-six in 2006 after crashing his experimental aircraft into the ocean just off the coast of Wilmington, North Carolina. Bracey was a thrill seeker; whether it was water skiing—he was the best water skier on our home lake of Lake James—snow skiing, or any other sport I witnessed him enjoy over the years, Bracey seemed indestructible. But I knew in my heart that Bracey's risks would eventually be what did him in. Unfortunately, I was right.

At any rate, Dr. Jacobs was someone I came to rely on. He explained at every step where I was in my recovery. He confirmed things that I had suspected. It was comforting to have his guidance through this long time of uncertainty. He was forthright in that he could make no predictions about my recovery time. So little research had been done on Guillain-Barré that my improvement would largely be determined by my body's response to the treatment. My treatment consisted of various medications and equipment. I was hooked to a party of hanging IV bags and a feeding tube, but the most important piece of equipment was a ventilator that breathed on my behalf. My lungs had completely shut down, and I relied on the ventilator to live. The reliance on the ventilator became an obsession for me, resulting in a myriad of vivid dreams.

Dr. Jacobs made it clear that getting well was up to me. I had no problem with this. I figured that since I had gotten this far, losing was not an option. Again, I had faith in my upbringing and life experience thus far.

CHAPTER TWO

A NOD TOWARD RECOVERY

Doctor Jacobs was one of many medical professionals I came to know during my two months at St. Joseph's. About two years after leaving St. Joseph's, I went back to visit them on the LTAC floor, and I was surprised at how many remembered me. Some recalled my name—but they all recalled my room number. I guess that's the easiest way to remember a patient because in your day-to-day duties as a healthcare professional, names are always changing, but the room numbers stay the same.

I'd noticed the same thing in the prison system. Employees, especially frontline employees, nearly always responded the same way when asked about a particular inmate. They'd immediately recall the inmate's cell number, rarely calling a prisoner by name. In the hospital I became 4 or *404*.

An especially pleasing thing I encountered on my return visit that day was that each of them smiled when they saw me. I fondly remember the day I was discharged from St. Joseph's.

Dr. Jacobs told me, "There sure are going to be a lot of girls here who hate to see you go, but remember that they are happy for you." All the smiles I saw when I visited two years later removed any doubt that he might have been just pumping me up.

Let me explain what Dr. Jacobs meant. The word that stands out to me is *girls*. If you've ever spent much time in a hospital, then you know that they are operated primarily by women. Yes, a disproportionate number of the doctors and surgeons are male; but by and large, hospitals are operated by females. And that was just fine with me. I've always been a ladies' man, but during my illness, it was different. It's hard to flirt when you're lying on your back, paralyzed, and utterly vulnerable with a breathing machine taking every breath for you.

Setting aside the flirting and ladies' man stuff, I've always enjoyed the company of women much more than that of men. Don't get me wrong, I like being around my buddies as much as the next guy; but for quality time—especially conversation—I prefer women. I think they're more honest, caring, sincere, and most of all (drum roll please), more intelligent than men. If you could look at my Facebook friends list, you would find that about three-quarters of them are women. I discovered this preference at a fairly early age. Being around women just made me feel better than being around guys.

Now before anybody starts jumping to incorrect conclusions, let me be very clear—I am about as far from being a homosexual as one can be. I just love women.

For all intents and purposes, if you enjoy the company of women and have confidence in the care they can provide to you, you're in a better position if you are hospitalized.

One loss that was difficult to come to grips with—and this became most evident while I was at St. Joseph's because I was finally conscious and aware of my surroundings again—was my loss of pride. It's one thing to be undressed by your lover during a romantic encounter; it's a completely different feeling when it's an activity of daily living that you should be able to accomplish by yourself, you have no say-so in the matter, and it's being carried out by women whose names you can only read on a nametag. It took a great deal of getting used to, but as time wore on, I was able to accept their help without feeling shame.

The staff on the LTAC floor were exceptional. Right from the start I got a true feeling of caring from all of them. Their attitude and behavior made this chapter of the adventure easier to handle.

Sometimes when I tell my story, I make light of certain events. This is a coping mechanism, a way to handle my reflection on what was a very dark period. When I had just come out of six weeks of hovering between life and death—even though it appeared unlikely that I would die—it was uncertain whether I would recover from the paralysis and overcome the dependence on machines for survival.

It's disconcerting when your thoughts are all you have, twenty-four hours a day. Sleep, receiving care, and the occasional visitor were my only distractions. That left about sixteen hours every day to think; and believe me, they aren't all good thoughts that pop into your mind. I often wished I was sedated again so I wouldn't have to deal with thoughts of *What if?* The care I received, coupled with my own perseverance, gradually diminished these thoughts, especially when I started seeing bits of improvement.

Dr. Jacobs came into my room each day during his daily rounds and, after saying "Good morning," he'd walk to the foot of my bed, squeeze one of my toes, and ask if I could feel anything. Invariably, I would shake my head. Every morning it was the same thing, squeeze a toe, ask me the question—and I would shake my head. In an odd way, I came to look forward to this morning meeting. I couldn't speak and couldn't move except for my head, but at least I could communicate on some level—and even if the communication was always the same, I had control over something. It was the way I started my day, and the redundancy was grounding, creating a normalcy that calmed me.

Remember what I said at the beginning of this story about always taking a shower in the same manner and the same order each morning? I have always been superstitious, and veering from routine bothers me.

So, to start my day with a new, simple routine made me feel more in my element. With all the madness running through my mind, anything that returned me to expectations of day-to-day life was reassuring. It made me feel as if I was in control a little bit and that I was part of my own recovery plan.

Each day started the same. I could see the clock on the wall and anticipate the staff's shift change. I observed their daily routines and—if I had been able to speak—I could probably have told you better than they could have explained it themselves what they'd be doing at a certain time. Anything that went on inside my room, in the hallway, or in the corner of the nurses' station that I could see from my bed became my entertainment. In a strange way, my prison career had prepared me for this task. One of your biggest responsibilities as a correctional employee is to observe behavior. That's what you do all day, every day. You observe behavior and note anything that deviates from normal activity. If you do it long enough and you pay this activity the attention it deserves, you can become quite the expert.

Anything happening in my line of sight became etched in my mind. I became so observant that if one of the nurses wasn't feeling well or was having a bad day, I sensed it before her co-workers did. I couldn't do a damn thing about it, but I could pick up on it. There were so many times I wanted to ask, "Hey, what's wrong? Are you not feeling well? Can I help? Do you want someone to talk to?" But I couldn't. It was disheartening, but I kept telling myself that the day would come when I would be able to voice my thoughts again.

One day, things started out as they normally did. The first-shift staff took over at the regular time. I noted which rotation was working—they always seemed to group the same people together. This was another thing we did in the prison. All uniformed staff were assigned to specific shifts and rotations, which changed only on rare occasions when someone from another rotation had to fill in. We formed a camaraderie and reliance on our team members. Teamwork aided in confidence-building and set in motion a smoother operation with fewer mistakes. The hospital setting operated in the same manner. Dr. Jacobs wasn't assigned to a rotation but generally worked an 8-to-5 schedule—the same way that management staff worked in the prison. On this particular day, he walked into my room as he had all the other days, said, "Good morning, Danny," picked out a toe, squeezed it, and asked if I could feel anything. I looked straight at him—and nodded my head.

My God! I could actually feel him squeezing my toe! I was elated and shocked at the same time. I hadn't expected this. I was ecstatic. I thought, *Well I sure didn't see that coming, but by God I'm sure glad it did!* It was that feeling multiplied by about a million. I couldn't laugh or even smile. I couldn't cry or even look shocked. I couldn't yell or scream—all of which I wanted to do after so many weeks of the complete absence of feeling anywhere in my body. All these emotions exploded in my mind at this exact moment.

The day I had kept telling myself would come, had finally arrived. *Hurray, hurray, hurray!* I finally had something tangible that I could hold in my mind and on which I could build the rest of my recovery.

This had to be the start of some real improvement.

Some kind of return to normal.

Some sort of end to the unbelievable—and a return to the believable.

I will never forget that moment. Such a small, insignificant act had manifested itself into one of the biggest accomplishments of my life! I wish there had been a camera in my room to record the moment for posterity. Hell, I wish there had been a news crew on hand so it could have made the evening news. "Well Ted, I'm happy to report that Danny was finally able to feel a doctor squeeze his toe today, and he nodded his head to acknowledge it. Film at 11."

One small sensation in one little toe was all I needed to begin my journey back to myself.

CHAPTER THREE

HONOR AMONG THIEVES

The year was 1998 and I had recently been promoted to Sergeant at the prison. On Tuesdays we shipped out and received inmates. These transfers occurred for various reasons: security, inmate requests, program availability, institutional needs, and the like. Once in a while we would receive a high-profile inmate. They were classified as such because of a crime the inmate had committed in society—or while incarcerated. This particular inmate was classified as high profile due to the former.

His name was Daniel Andre Green, and he, along with his crime partner, Larry Demery, had murdered a gentleman by the name of James Jordan in Lumberton, North Carolina. The reason the crime was high profile was because of who James Jordan's son was—none other than basketball superstar Michael Jordan. *The* Michael Jordan.

I was notified that Green would be assigned to my unit. We were always notified ahead of time so we could take precautions. In Green's case, he'd been in prison only a short time and nothing out of the ordinary had occurred in regard to him. I notified my officers at the beginning of the shift that he'd be transferring in but gave no further instructions except to keep their eyes and ears open and let me know if anything unusual happened.

Michael Jordan was a hero to a lot of inmates, just as he was to many members of the general public. He was perhaps adored even more so because our entire inmate population was male, and a tremendous number of inmates are intensely focused on athletics. Sports becomes their outlet, either through participation or observation, as evidenced by the activity inside a housing wing when a key basketball or football game is on TV. Every set of eyes in that wing will be glued to the set. Also, just as it is on the street, sports is a major object of gambling in prison.

If you have an individual who has coldly murdered the father of a hero of a population of men housed in an atmosphere where they don't wish to be, you have a recipe for disaster. You also have to remember that these men are in this atmosphere for actions a bit more severe than singing too loudly in the church choir. But again, so far, so good.

Green was escorted back to my unit just as many others were every week. He was assigned to our only open cell: one on the mezzanine. We had two levels on each floor, and the mezzanine was on top. The sergeant's office was located on the same floor—not on the mezzanine, but still in close proximity. Green was placed in the cell with a short introduction about our schedule and what was expected of him. It was the regular routine, and we all went about our business. He arrived after the evening meal when inmate activity usually slowed to a crawl, which it did on this day.

Suddenly, things changed rapidly.

Around 7:00 p.m. I got up from my desk to walk toward the back gate. I didn't get two steps when a loud banging on the observation glass got my attention. The inmates know not to beat on the glass; so when I heard it, I was concerned, especially since it came from Green's wing.

I turned to see an inmate pointing and yelling, "Sarge, you gotta help him!" I looked into the wing to see an inmate face down on the floor at the bottom of the mezzanine stairwell. I ordered the wing door opened and rushed over. It was Daniel Green. I asked him if he was alright and got no response other than a couple of grunts. Reaching down to turn his head toward me, I discovered massive wounds to his face. He had gotten the shit beat out of him. I asked him how it happened, but he didn't answer.

I asked the inmate who had first alerted me. He told me that Green had slipped and fallen. Clearly that was a crock of bull. I immediately radioed for medical assistance, notified my officer in charge (OIC), and ordered the wing locked down.

While I waited for them to arrive, I kept trying to get Green to talk to me; but he said nothing. Once the medical personnel had completed preliminary treatment on Green, he was sent with EMS to the local hospital. I walked up to Green's cell and called to have the door opened. I walked in and saw blood splatters as well as an obvious disarray of clothing and linens. There was no doubt that he'd been assaulted inside his cell.

At the time, cameras had been installed only in key areas of the institution; housing areas weren't included. Therefore, we had no one to rely on for witness accounts other than the inmates in that wing. No staff had observed the incident. It had been my experience that sooner or later an inmate informant, a snitch, would come forward. This was especially true when an assault had occurred. I guess the inmates look at it as we do in society. If I know who assaulted someone in my neighborhood, I'd better inform law enforcement because I—or a member of my family—may very well be the next victim. Prisons operate in pretty much the same manner, even though it may be more difficult to get a witness to come forward.

We questioned every inmate in the wing individually and in private, but no one would talk. The story we kept getting was either, "I didn't see anything," or "He just fell down the stairs." Sometimes it takes several days before a snitch will talk. Sometimes he's waiting for the perfect time or for the right person to feel safe talking.

Eventually, one inmate was named in the assault. The reason was said to be retribution for a gambling debt at another institution where the two had been housed together. While the story felt false, it's the one we had to go with. As a result, the assailant was charged and served a lengthy time in segregation for the assault. Two or three years later, I finally heard an account of the incident that I feel was truthful. I heard that the "assailant" had volunteered to take the heat for the assault and was later paid for his actions by the other inmates. They wanted our staff to stop investigating the incident to end the increased observation and pressure on the wing. This story also made it clear that the assault had occurred for the reason I thought it did. The inmates wanted to mess up the guy who had killed their hero's father. Maybe there's honor among thieves after all.

CHAPTER FOUR

LESSONS IN LOSING

I believe my involvement in athletics growing up helped me tremendously during my recovery from Guillain-Barré. I've heard many times that the greatest lesson one learns through participation in sports during your formative years is to put forth the required effort needed to obtain your goal—to win. While this may be true for some, I believe the greatest lesson from playing sports is that it teaches you how to lose. This is especially true in baseball, where the sheer number of games played presents you with more opportunities to lose.

In my opinion, handling a win is no challenge whatsoever. "Hooray, we won! Everything is right with the world! Everybody's happy! No problem! We came out ahead!" You can't go wrong with winning. It goes over great every time.

Losing, on the other hand, is a different matter. And losing will come to you in life just as does in athletics. How you handle loss makes all the difference in how you approach the next game.

In baseball you're considered an excellent hitter if you achieve a batting average of .300 or better. That means you were able to get a base hit at least three times out of every ten opportunities you had. Just think about that. Three times out of every ten chances you're successful, and seven times you fail. But you're still considered an excellent hitter.

One of my favorite quotes comes from a baseball movie, *Bull Durham,* when Ebby Calvin "Nuke" LaLoosh (Tim Robbins) responds to an interview question by saying, "Sometimes you win, sometimes you lose, sometimes it rains."

Life often mirrors this mindset. In life you always want to win; but inevitably, you're going to fail a large part of the time. Sometimes these failures can be attributed directly to something you did, but many times you have no power whatsoever to convert that failure into a success. Shit happens.

I believe that the earlier in life you learn to deal with losing, the better off you are. That's one reason I detest the widely held practice of presenting trophies to all the participants in an event—whether they did anything remarkable or not. Participation carries its own award, and receiving a prize for doing your job sends the wrong message. Winners deserve recognition for having succeeded, and it takes away from their accomplishments to reward the losers.

My first failure on the field had a profound effect on me, and what I learned from it stayed with me.

It was 1969. I was ten years old, and Nebo was getting its first Little League Baseball team together. The age range was ten to thirteen, so I was barely old enough to try out. My father had been working with me to learn the various aspects of the game for two years, and I was eager to finally play on a team. He and I practiced when he got home from working in the cotton mill every day. I also learned some during recess in school, when we played softball pickup games in the neighborhood, and during the structured recreation programs that

Coach Richard Laney organized during the summer for all the kids in town.

The first tryout day was held on a Saturday morning. We split up according to the positions we were interested in playing. All the kids got a chance to field a few batted balls from one of the coaches, and then we all took some swings during batting practice. Everything went pretty well for me for the first two activities. It was the next exercise that spelled trouble. We were told to run two laps all the way around the edge of the field and meet back at home plate.

Now, here's where you should know that, even though I was in pretty good athletic shape for a ten-year-old kid, I was a few pounds overweight—so distance running was not my forte. When the second lap came around, I was completely out of breath. By the time I got to the right field area, I stopped running and started to walk home. In addition to being disappointed, I was greatly embarrassed. The worst criticism, however, came after I got home. When my father asked me how it had gone at the tryout, I told him the truth. I'll never forget the look of disappointment on his face when he said, "After all the work we put in after work every day in the backyard, and you quit. I just don't understand."

Those words hurt me more than anything else I remember up to that point in my life. The embarrassment I felt paled in comparison to my heartache when I realized just how much I had disappointed my father. I swore that day that I would never allow this to happen again for the rest of my life, and I never did.

The events of that day taught me valuable lessons—lessons that can't be learned from a book or in a classroom. Lessons that can only be learned from life and having lost.

CHAPTER FIVE

PROGRESS LITTLE BY LITTLE

Well, with at least a little feeling back in my toe, I thought my recovery should speed up—and it did. Little by little— and oh, I do mean little by little—things did start to improve. After a few more days, I was able to achieve a tiny bit of movement in a couple of my fingers. That, along with a slight ability to move my arms, was huge. It might sound silly, but my focus was on being able to point and wave again. Let me explain why.

Like every other thing I had lost during this misadventure, I never realized how much something means to me until it's not there anymore. It's kind of like letting a personal rela-tionship fall apart that you really didn't think was all that at the time. A relationship with the potential to turn into some-thing you'd give anything to have back a little ways down the road. It's the same thing I found out in regard to simple bodily operations.

We learn to point and wave at a very early age. We learn to point to indicate where our interest lies at that moment, and wave to acknowledge our fellow man. There's no voice needed because we learn to communicate these things before we learn to speak.

That's exactly what I faced; learning to do most everything without having the ability to speak. You don't need to talk when you're trying to focus all your energy on simple tasks again.

Looking back on the entire story, Guillain-Barré took me back to being an infant, except with an adult's mind. One day I was a normal, healthy, fully functioning adult male. The next I found myself paralyzed, but still able to communicate verbally. A few days later, I lost the ability to speak, and they told me that the only known treatment hadn't worked. There was no way to predict what would happen next, and it could— and almost certainly would—get worse.

Then I was told in a roundabout way that I may be facing death. No one ever said it outright, but my mind still worked, and I'm no idiot, so I figured out the gist of their messages. I remember thinking that I might just find out what it's like to die.

A couple of days later I was sedated.

The day came when I woke up to be told it appeared the worst was over. It really was like being born again, but not in the biblical sense. After fifty-six years I was experiencing a second birth. Thank goodness this time I didn't shit all over myself.

Each day became an adventure in trying to learn how to do basic things again. I'd wake up and think, *Hey let's see what might start to move today. Let's see where I might be able to feel something again.* Some days progressed better than others, and some days I regressed. It's still that way today.

I never know when I go to bed at night just how much feeling or mobility I'll have in my feet when I wake up. I've tried to find a common denominator, considering my activities or diet, from a day when I feel good as opposed to a day when I'm in more pain, but nothing adds up. There's no way to predict how bad the neuropathy in my feet will be, how intense the tingling in my fingertips will be, or just how much my total mobility will be hindered.

This is frustrating as hell. Before my crisis, I didn't have to think about planning ahead for my physical well-being just to go out for a day—or even an hour. Those days are gone. Instead of planning where I would spend a fun weekend, planning ahead now covers pretty much each step I'm going to take to get from point A to point B on any given day. I can plan activities, but there's no guarantee that I'll be able to carry them out.

My planning has been magnified to a degree that I never expected. When we go through life unhindered physically, we effortlessly plan for activities—days, weeks, months, or even years in the future—relatively certain that physical limitations won't hold us back. For me, planning is now a minute-to-minute exercise. I can envision participating, but I'm not very confident that I'll be able to take part as I wish. My plans change often instead of rarely these days. This can be frustrating, but I won't let it destroy my life. It may hinder, but it will not destroy. As time wears on, we all can get used to nearly anything if it occurs often enough; and believe me, what I've just described occurs every day.

There were a couple of stints when I worked in a cotton mill. Cotton mills take in raw materials such as cotton, Dacron, and polyester, in one end of the plant; and after it goes through various means of processing, it comes out the other end of the plant as fabric. Cotton mills were a major employer in the south during the last century, but they've all but completely disappeared from the landscape because nearly all the fabric we use in the U.S. today is produced abroad. Even though it's manufactured at a lower cost overseas, I feel the main reason this industry has vanished from modern-day America is that cotton mill work is tough manual labor—and today's American workforce is unwilling to put in the effort required. In other words, today's workers couldn't tie the shoes of the average American worker from my parents' generation.

Cotton mill work was hard, hot, dirty physical labor. I found this out firsthand. It was divided into three eight-hour shifts, which normally operated six days per week. I worked third shift, 11:00 PM to 7:00 AM. I'd always bring an extra T-shirt with me to work, as the one I had on would be completely soaked after a couple of hours. I'd change into a dry one and hang the wet one up to dry, repeating this sequence through the night. Two things surprised me about cotton mill work: one, the level of hard physical labor required to do the job; and two, there were no windows. When your shift started you belonged to the mill. It had a hold on you that, no matter how hard you wanted to, you couldn't break until shift change. It was then, and only then, that you could breathe fresh air again and take in whatever view lay outside the door.

Both my parents were career cotton mill employees. It wasn't until I went to work in the mill that I came to appreciate their work discipline. As I stated before, the mill operated six days per week, and you were expected to be there every day. There was no sick time or vacation time in those days. You didn't show up for work—you didn't get paid. Simple as that. No ifs, ands, or buts about it. The mill closed for one week over July 4th, and that was it. If you wanted another week off, you had to quit your job to get it.

The only time I ever remember my mom being off work was when she was either about to give birth or when she was nursing a newborn—and as soon as that newborn was weaned, it was back to work for Mama. My dad's work record was even more impressive. Daddy worked the same job in the mill for a grand total of forty-seven years and retired with forty-seven years of perfect attendance. That's right; he worked nearly a half century without missing a day. I've never forgotten the work ethic of my parents, and I believe it's a major contributing factor in the person I turned out to be—and I'm proud of that.

Getting back to the frustration of learning new tasks and essentially being reduced to being a baby again, there's one huge difference. A baby's mind doesn't already know how to perform these tasks. Mine already did. A baby just tries to imitate what it observes going on around it. Failure means nothing. It has never succeeded, so there's no way it can fail. It can only try to do what it sees others doing.

My mind not only knew how to perform these tasks, it had also been conditioned over the years to avoid failure. Before Guillain-Barré, I didn't experience failure often; and if I did, I could correct the problem quickly. But after Guillain-Barré, failure was constant. Success was scarce. This was good and bad. It was good that it drove me harder to succeed, but it was bad in that constant failure made giving up a viable option.

I decided early on that failure would not be an option. Remember the old saying, "I'll make it or die trying"? That was pretty much the mindset I adopted. I'm going to live my life as I want, or I might as well be dead; and I was going to do everything in my power to remain as alive as I could be. That's all there was to it.

As I mentioned before, being able to speak wasn't essential to learning basic tasks again, but by golly, it sure didn't make it any easier. Being unable to speak may have been the most frustrating aspect of the whole adventure, and there wasn't a damn thing I could do about it—or was there?

As I slowly regained the ability to use my fingers to point, one day it occurred to me that if I had something with the alphabet on it nearby, I could point to the letters of the words that I wanted so badly to speak. I could articulate, nonverbally, what was on my mind. I can't remember exactly how I got this idea across to anyone, but it happened one day when a nurse showed me one of my get-well cards. This wasn't an everyday occurrence, but a lot of my friends went to the trouble of sending me cards, which was incredibly helpful to my mindset. The nurses would tell me who had sent a card, read it to me, and then pin it onto my bulletin board where just the sight of the cards gave me hope and confidence.

One day as a nurse read me a card, I somehow got her to open it and hold it closer to me. I pointed to a word; she said the word and looked quizzically at me. I kept pointing at one letter in the word—and eventually she said the letter instead of the word. I nodded emphatically. *Yes!* This was a huge step, and in no time, they had a legal pad with all the letters of the alphabet and the numbers from 0 to 9 on it right there at my bed. I could suddenly, at a rudimentary level—and with the help of a nurse or CNA with a pen—speak again!

I remember many staff members coming in and getting a kick out of seeing how I was able to communicate by pointing at letters to create the words that I wanted so badly to roll off my tongue. Every single person who walked into room 404 and saw what we had figured out broke into an ear-to-ear smile; and if I had been able to form a smile at that point I would have joined right in. Unfortunately, smiling was still a little ways down the road. Even though I couldn't break into a smile on the outside, believe me, I sure was smiling on the inside. This progress bolstered my confidence. Finally, there was something tangible in my physical and mental progress.

A couple of days later, one of the nurses took it one step further and walked in with a dry erase board and a couple of pens. Brilliant! Why didn't I think of that? We no longer had to keep flipping pages on the legal pad. Just wipe off what I had already said and move on to the next words. It was like a game that I didn't want to stop playing. Even so, it did get frustrating when I couldn't remember how to spell a word, or when the stopping point for a word was misunderstood by whoever was attempting to make out words from the letters I pointed at with a wavering finger. Even with all the frustration, the result was worth it for me. I think it was worth it for the nurses as well. They really did seem to get satisfaction from seeing my happiness.

I've included a picture taken around this time of me lying in my bed with the dry erase board beside my head showing the phrase, "Happy Thanksgiving to all of you. Danny." Look closely and you can see the slightest semblance of a smile around my mouth, as well as a little twinkle in my eyes. Everything seemed to be improving. The photo was taken by my friend Duane just before the holiday. Thanksgiving had always been my favorite holiday. Over the previous several years at work, I would cut a deal with my assistant—giving

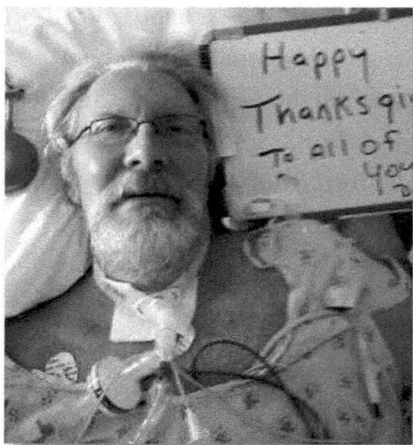

Danny's memorable Thanksgiving,
St. Joseph's Hospital, Nov., 2015

him or her the week of Christmas off in exchange for my being able to take the week of Thanksgiving off. Obviously, this improvement happened at an auspicious time.

Duane posted the picture on my Facebook page to provide an update for all my friends. He always showed me the pictures he posted so I could see how many responses were attached to the photos. It would be several months later, when I was a patient in the rehab hospital, before I regained the dexterity to use my laptop and explore all the encouraging comments, soaking in each and every individual *Like* and *Love* icon left for me. People can say what they want about the downside of social media—and there definitely is a downside—but I can assure you that reading all that encouragement on Facebook helped this fellow more than you can imagine. We can get a little cynical and jaded, especially as we grow older. I've always tried to avoid this, but it still happens. It was amplified during my twenty years in a prison environment. When you're surrounded by negativity 95 percent of the time, being jaded feels like your natural state. The support I felt from everyone through these Facebook updates reduced my cynicism and renewed my faith in my fellow man. I guess there are some caring people left in the world. I never imagined I had so many friends.

CHAPTER SIX

JONNA

I was lucky enough to be visited by many friends. However, I was not prepared for one of the visits I received around Thanksgiving.

Back in the '80s when I was in the music business, mixing sound and road managing the band Passenger, I met a girl named Jonna Robol from the Norfolk/Virginia Beach area— our band's hottest territory. Jonna and I hit it off from the first time we laid eyes on each other, and we ended up living together in a Virginia Beach townhouse during '85 and '86. When the band broke up and came off the road in the summer of '86, Jonna and I decided to go our

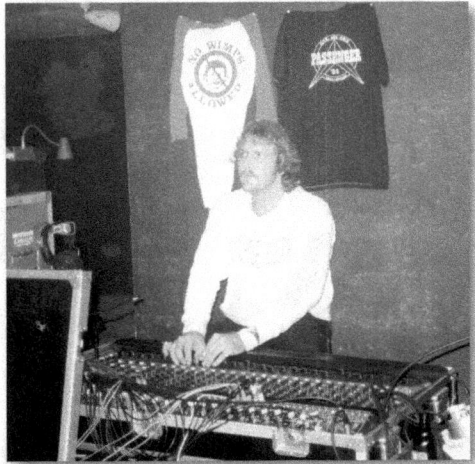

Danny at sound board, Passenger concert, circa 1983

separate ways as well. She remained in the area, as she had grown up there; but I moved back to Nebo. Jonna got married and had a child named Cortney. But the marriage didn't last long, and by 1991 she and I had rekindled our friendship.

For several years, at least once a year and often at Thanksgiving, I'd travel back to the Tidewater area to spend a few days with Jonna and Cortney. They would also travel to North Carolina to spend a few days with me occasionally. After Cortney had grown up and gone off to college, Jonna and I continued to see each other when we could. We talked on a regular basis. We attended many events through the years, and we even managed to ring in the new millennium together in Charlotte, North Carolina.

Lo and behold, lying in that hospital bed one day, I looked up—and there stood Jonna, along with one of our friends, Chris. I remember thinking I was having another one of those

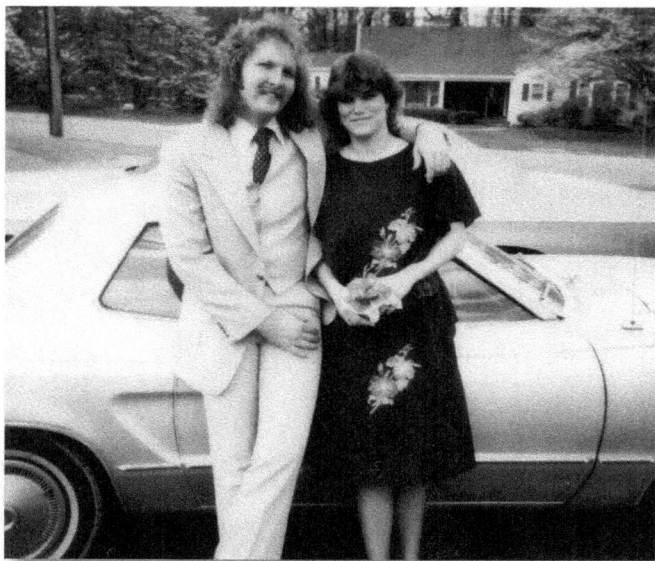

Danny and Jonna, wedding of our drummer, Statesville, NC, 1984

wild dreams (I'll tell you about those later), wondering, *Are they really here?* Well, they really were there—right in front of me. Jonna had contacted my brother, and the two of them planned to visit me and stay at my house. I couldn't have gotten a better gift for Thanksgiving. One of the most special friends of my entire life was standing right there looking down at me in my hospital bed. She and Chris had driven over 300 miles to check on their old friend who was having it rough. I couldn't have received a better gift in any way, shape, form, or fashion. The hits just kept on coming!

When I talked to Jonna several months later, I asked her impression of seeing me in the condition I was in. It was hard for me even to say the words *paralyzed, half-dead*, and *limp*. I wasn't a version of myself I ever imagined to be, especially so helpless in front of her.

The first thing out of her mouth was that it hurt her to see my frustration to communicate with her—or anyone else, for that matter.

She has no idea how right she was. I was excited beyond belief to see her and Chris. I wanted to reach out and hug her. But I couldn't do that. Kiss her. Couldn't do that. Hold her hand. Couldn't do that. Speak to her. Couldn't do even that. The only thing I could do was write on the board. However, I guess my adrenaline was pumping so hard that it made me speed up an arduous process. I was impatient to see my thoughts written on that dry erase board and expressed to her, but it wasn't like speaking with her.

Jonna and I had our differences through the years, but one thing we never had a problem with was talking. Even when we weren't together, we would talk on the phone for hours. I can't tell you how many times we'd been 400 miles apart, talking on the phone until the wee hours. And then, during the most trying, devastating time in my life, we were face to face and I couldn't speak the first word.

My frustration was amplified because I'd regained the use of some of my facial muscles, making it easier to read my feelings just by looking at my face. I tried my best to put on a brave, confident front, but I'm sure she saw through it.

On the other hand, Jonna and Chris had come to see me, and they were expecting the worst. My brother has a way of seeing the worst-case scenario in a situation, and he was the one who had relayed to them the information regarding my condition. So, I'm sure they were relieved to see that ol' Dan wasn't quite standing on death's doorstep after all. Gosh, I didn't want to see them leave. I valued every visit during that period, but there was only one other that reached the level of satisfaction that this one brought—I'll get to it later.

By this time, I had gotten used to not being able to eat anything. By this point, I could move my head and upper torso far enough to actually see that ugly bag of sustenance if I put some effort into it. Day after day I'd look up at that bag hanging there, containing my breakfast, lunch, and dinner— or *supper* as it's referred to in the South. I had no ability to ask for a snack, but I really would have loved to have some peanuts, potato chips, pig skins, popcorn . . . anything. But I couldn't.

Oh, how I missed the taste of spaghetti, beef and gravy, mashed potatoes, a really good steak—the list could go on forever, but it paled in comparison to the agony of not being able to enjoy another one of life's pleasures, actually one of its necessities.

Drinking!

We must take in some sort of liquid on a regular basis or we'll die. The average time I think a human can live without liquids is about four days. The simplest thing for a human to drink is, of course, water. In the United States, the options for beverages are seemingly endless. There is tea, coffee, milk, beer, wine, liquor, and ten thousand soft drinks. All of these drinks have one thing in common. The base ingredient is water. Common, simple water. It's usually available quite readily. I've always been a big water drinker. Being involved in athletics growing up, we were encouraged to stay hydrated. "Drink more water!" Good, sound advice. You can't go wrong drinking more water for better health. Trust me, I didn't have to be encouraged. I loved the stuff, and the water from my well at home—the same well I still drink from every day—is the best-tasting water I've ever had. Some say water has no taste. I say you've never had water from my well. Good old Nebo water. The finest in the world. So, it would stand to reason that if this essential drink was denied to a water lover such as myself, it would be unnerving. Well, that's exactly how it was.

When I was initially placed on a ventilator, a tube was inserted into my neck at the meeting of the collar bones—you know, that little place under your Adam's apple that leads down into your chest. With it, a feeding tube was introduced into my torso just below my left rib cage; my ability to take in food and drink through my mouth came to a sudden end. Being intubated allowed me to keep breathing, and therefore keep living, even without my lungs operating on their own. That's a great thing, but intubation had a definite downside: I could aspirate should I take in liquid through my mouth too rapidly. I had heard of aspiration but didn't really know the definition. Once I was conscious again, they explained that if I took in fluids too quickly through my mouth while on a ventilator, I would choke to death. As a result, my fluid intake was restricted and monitored closely.

Forget drinking water; my only fluid intake was ice chips, which were fed to me from a Styrofoam cup on a plastic spoon by a nurse about every thirty minutes while I was awake. I said earlier that you can get used to almost anything after a while. I did not get used to this.

Not long after Jonna and Chris's visit, I had improved to the point that they started weening me off the ventilator so I could depend on my lungs again. As with everything else, this major leap started with tiny steps. The breathing tube was removed from where it had been inserted at the base of my neck. At first, they left it out for just seconds, slowly increasing the time I breathed on my own. Shortly, they could leave it out for minutes, then hours, and before long, for good!

My thirst wasn't intense until I was removed from the ventilator and regained the ability to speak. While this was definitely an improvement, it also made my thirst intensify. I guess being able to run my mouth caused it to dry out more quickly, increasing my craving.

CHAPTER SEVEN

SWALLOW TEST

We've all experienced thirst. I'd guess it's one of the first discomforts a baby realizes. How does a baby indicate that it's hungry or thirsty? It cries. And babies cry a lot. Water remains a deep need for life.

The first intense thirst I can remember happened when I was ten or eleven years old. During the summer, a lot of us neighborhood kids would get together for pickup baseball games at Nebo School. There was no water fountain at the field, not even a garden hose. One thing that we did have was a natural spring located down a hill about thirty yards below the field. When we got thirsty enough, we'd take a break and walk through the woods down to the spring and drink out of the pipe that delivered water from God-only-knows how far underground. Man, that was good water—and always cold! The only problem was that, by the time you made the hike back up the hill through the woods to the ballfield, you'd be thirsty again. One day, one of the guys showed up with a Pepsi, which only came in ten-ounce glass bottles back then. He was smart enough to save the empty bottle. When we took our first break, he carried the bottle down to the spring, and right before we made the trek back up the hill, he filled the bottle with water and carried it back so he'd have water back on the field. Genius! From that day on, an empty bottle or cup of some sort became part of the essential gear we took to the baseball field. Glove, check. Ball, check. Bat, check. Cap, check. Something with which to carry water back from the spring and up the hill, check!

All the times I'd ever experienced thirst in my life paled in comparison to what I experienced in the hospital. The feeling was the same. The arid, parched, almost leathery feel inside my mouth and on my lips was identical. The difference came with the realization that an end was not in sight. A quenching of that thirst was not just a matter of minutes or hours away. I was unable to get that wonderful, delightful feeling of a cold beverage flowing over my tongue and down my throat. I had no way to achieve satisfaction. And one of the worst parts about it was that the very people who had kept me alive and cared for me were the same ones keeping me from gaining this satisfaction.

Believe me, I tried my best to talk them into it. I got to the point of begging. Humility had left town long ago. If begging is what it took, then so be it. I took advantage of every staff member who walked into 404. I hoped at least one of them would feel sorry enough for me to give me a few sips of water. What could that hurt? Maybe I could convince more than one of them to give in. I kissed every ass that walked into that room before starting my sob story for the day. Someone was bound to cave.

Wrong. They stuck together. I was never able to uncover a traitor, despite my best efforts. However, just a couple of days after kissing that ventilator goodbye forever, one of these disciplined people came to me with the information I'd been waiting to hear. Her name was Alisha, and she was the first-shift head nurse that day. Alisha and I had established a good relationship, and the news I got from her on that day led to a memory that I will carry with me for the rest of my life. She told me she was taking me downstairs for a swallow test.

My response was, "What the hell is a swallow test?"

She answered, "It's something that you've been waiting for, for a very long time."

Hmm, this sounds interesting. Let's do it. She wheeled my bed (with the IV rack leashed to me) out of my room and over to the elevator. We went down a couple of floors to a new area of the hospital, new to me anyway. Several nurses waited there for us. They explained that a swallow test is just what the name implies: a test to see if my system could swallow without choking.

Several monitors were attached to my midsection. They were also connected to instruments behind a glass partition in an adjacent room. I'd be given a series of foods to chew and swallow normally to see if I could keep them down.

Again, here's my comparison to an infant. When a baby stops nursing and starts eating, you feed it foods with different consistencies to find out what it can tolerate. Once more, I was in baby mode.

The first thing they gave me was applesauce. Someone placed a small spoonful in my mouth. I chewed it, or at least rolled it around in my mouth, actually tasting food for the first time in a long while. I didn't want to swallow it for two reasons: Number one, I didn't want to possibly fail the test.

Number two, I relished the taste. Just think about it. I hadn't had food of any kind in my mouth in nearly four months.

Well, I did finally swallow it and voila! No problem. The test food intensified as far as texture was concerned. One after the next, I was able to get each of them down and keep them down with no problem. Then it came time for the final item. A plain saltine cracker. Dry, crunchy, and something that would go down in bigger pieces. This was quite a challenge, but I was determined to chew this thing up, swallow it, keep it down, and win the game. They placed the cracker in my mouth. I chewed it up as well as I could, opened up my throat, and sent it on its way. It felt as if it had worked fine to me, but my attention was on the two women monitoring the equipment behind the glass. After just a few seconds I saw each of them smile and give a thumbs up. Everyone gave me a round of applause and congratulated me! I could then be gradually placed back on a normal diet. Alisha wheeled me out of the area and back toward the elevator. But before we got there, she stopped and said she'd be right back. In a couple of minutes my friend Alisha brought me one of the greatest gifts I have ever received: a Coca-Cola on ice in a real glass. She told me that she'd watched me wishing to be able to drink something for so long, and she wanted to give me this because it hurt her to see me suffering.

She placed the rim of the glass up to my lips and gave me my first sip. My God, it tasted fantastic! She then asked if I thought I could hold the glass, and I said that I would sure give it a try. This was an adventure all on its own since my fingers were still curled up, but I pulled it off. I had been lucky enough to have the opportunities to drink excellent craft beers, fine wines, and expensive liquors, but let me tell you, that simple Coca-Cola was the best thing I've ever tasted. The ice-cold temperature. The slight stinging quality that a Coke has. The sweetness. Everything about it was as close as I can imagine to a heavenly experience.

The late, great, southern historian and humorist, Lewis Grizzard, once said that one of God's greatest creations was Coca-Cola. At that moment I was a true believer! I'll never forget that moment. I knew I was well on my way back to normal.

CHAPTER EIGHT

BEER LIKE WATER

Back in my band days, it wasn't unusual to drink beer pretty much anytime we could get it, and we could get it pretty much anytime we wanted to. Liquor rarely came into play if for no other reason than it was too expensive. But more likely it was just a lifestyle choice. All the road bands—and there were a lot, unlike today—drank beer like most people drink water, coffee, or juice. It just went along with the job. Drugs didn't come into the equation for the same reason that liquor didn't. They were too expensive. As I look back, the biggest

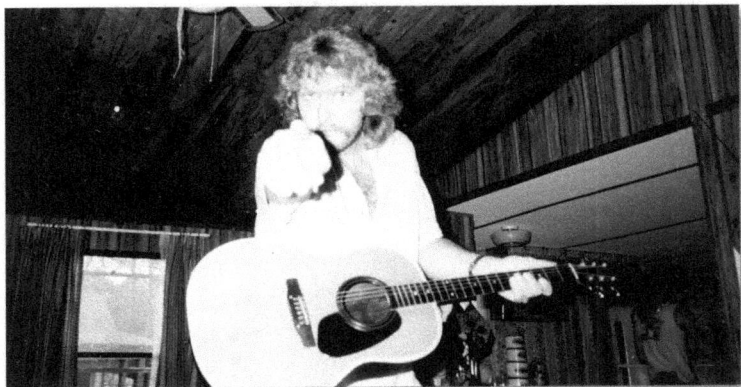

Fun on a rare day off the road, Charleston, SC, 1985

reason we drank beer was that it gave us a little high (but not too much) and allowed us to still do our job. For the most part, we weren't making a lot of money, and the work was hard—especially on setup days and tear-down nights. During the shows we had to keep our shit together, so getting drunk was not an option.

A special memory I'll always have is about my old road-buddy, Brian Watts. He often stayed in the same hotel room with me, especially during stretches when we had a lot of one nighters or other short duration jobs. During these jobs, I had to be ready to get the road crew going, usually early in the morning, plus do my road manager duties, and the guys on the crew had to be with me.

I can't tell you how many times I woke up in a hotel room, reached over to the nightstand, and grabbed a phonebook to identify which town it was, then reach for a beer. Brian and I kept a cooler on the floor between the beds so we could grab a beer first thing and get the day off to a productive start. On many occasions this was followed by turning on the TV and tuning in to *The Young and the Restless*. We had very little to anchor us to home on the road, and this seemed to help us in some strange way. That's how a lot of days started out back then, another example of how I always relied on something to drink as a core part of my routine.

CHAPTER NINE

MY FIRST DAY OF SCHOOL

My family moved from the small, close-knit manufacturing community of Clinchfield to the country-flavored, spread-out community of Nebo in late 1963. I had just turned five. Nebo was a rural area. There was no industry and, at that time, only a handful of small country stores. It had a post office, a volunteer fire department, and most importantly, its own school, which went from first grade all the way through high school.

There were three children in our family and my mother was expecting another by the time the beginning of school would roll around the next fall. I've already pointed out that both my parents had to work to provide for the family. This wasn't unusual, as the day of the homemaker was slowly eroding from the American family.

At the beginning of the school year, my mom chose to place me in first grade instead of waiting a year and starting at the usual age of six. You could get away with things like this back when everybody knew everybody else and things were simpler. I didn't know the difference. I just knew that my parents told me it was time to start school, so off I went. It wasn't until I was many years older that I realized that the majority of my classmates were a year older than I was. Not long before my mother passed away in 1997, she and I were talking one day and this subject came up. It had been no big deal to me while I was growing up, but on this day, I asked her why she had placed me in school early. She told me that with three kids about to become four, it was getting harder for her to raise us and keep her job. Remember how I stated earlier that shortly after I was weaned the neighborhood families had a large hand in raising me? In Nebo this wasn't practical because all the families lived far apart from each other. Besides, she said that she thought I was capable of handling it, so in late August of 1964, I was off to my first day of school.

We lived roughly a mile from the Nebo School, but I had no real idea where I lived in relation to it. Directions were things the adults were responsible for, not the type of thing a five-year-old little boy was concerned about.

The bus route passed right by our house and on the first day of school Mom sat on the front porch with me to await its arrival. I don't know why, but the events of that day have remained etched in my mind as if they happened just a few weeks ago instead of over fifty years ago. I can clearly remember the bus pulling up on the road in front of our house and stopping at the bottom of the driveway.

The bus, as I would soon find out, was the only snubnosed bus at Nebo School. Bus number thirty-nine. It was painted yellow like all the other buses but resembled a Trailways or Greyhound bus more than a regular school bus. Mom walked me to the end of the driveway, hugged me, told me to make her proud, and sent me on my way. I climbed up the wide, steep three or four steps (they were huge to a five-year-old kid), found a seat, and sat down among the other kids. I didn't know a one of those kids that day, but I'd quickly get to know almost all of them, as our neighborhood was a great place to grow up. Everybody got along well, and the general quality of life in small neighborhoods was so much safer and more open than it is today. Everybody knew everybody else. Everybody trusted everybody else and it was a better environment in which to grow up back in those days.

I had never been on a bus and I was fascinated by it. The sound of the big engine; a door that split in half and swung open when the driver moved a big, long handle; windows split in half that slid up and down; and it was so big that it had an aisle down the middle covered with rubber so we could walk between the seats. Amazing!

After a short drive, we arrived at school. The buses pulled around to the rear of the building to unload. A teacher was there when we got off the bus; and she had all of us first-graders stay with her, which was a good thing because we sure didn't know where we were or where we were going. Once we were all standing on solid ground again, she called off six or seven names, one of which was mine. She told us that at the end of the day we would not be taking bus thirty-nine home because it would be running a different route. We were to take bus number forty-nine.

Simple instructions, but not for a five-year-old. As the day progressed, my mind took in a myriad of new things. Sights, sounds, smells—everything was new. I was processing as much as possible and made new friends right off the bat. All in all, I was having a really good time. The whole day went smoothly. I remember thinking, *Hey, I think I'm really going to like this.* The end of the day came. Time to get back on the bus.

I'd forgotten the different bus number the teacher had given us that morning. You'd never know it today, but growing up, I was a bit shy—something that stuck with me for many years, causing trouble now and then. I was too shy to tell a grown up that I wasn't sure which bus I was supposed to take. So, rather than stand there and be left behind, I decided a good thing to do would be to get back on bus thirty-nine, the one that had brought me to this place. Surely it would return me to the other place I'd begun to like—my new home. It was easy enough to identify with its big flat front and giant size compared to the other buses. So, I got back on bus thirty-nine.

We rode around for a little while. The bus would stop and someone would get off. Sometimes more than one person got off. Sometimes it would be six or seven at a time. I remember thinking that some of these families sure must have a lot of kids!

Each time the bus stopped I looked out the window, but I didn't recognize any of the houses. So, I just kept riding and waiting to see my house through one of those funky windows split in half. The bus slowly emptied, and I never did see my house. I looked around and realized that I was the only person left. This kind of disturbed me, but I sat still, barely big enough to see over the back of the seat in front of me, with my mouth shut and my eyes open. Finally, the bus pulled off the road, went up a driveway, and parked. Back in those days, the buses were driven by high school students who took the buses home with them at night. At that moment, the driver got up from his seat and, scanning the seats, found me still sitting there. He then did one of those moves that one only does when totally frustrated. He placed his hand over his face and slowly pulled it down across his nose, lips, and chin, all the while letting out a very… long… sigh.

I thought my bus ride was over. It was not. He drove me back to the school. I was able to tell people my name, but I couldn't tell them where I lived because I really didn't know. We had just moved there. I couldn't provide them with a number to call because we didn't have a phone yet. I was stuck until they could figure out what to do with me. Eventually, along came a teacher who knew my mom, and she was able to give the principal directions to my house. Another kid had encountered the same problem on a different bus, so the principal put us both in his car and gave us a ride home.

One thing that stands out about this ride home was that the other kid—who was a year older than I was—cried the whole time. I never shed a tear. This lack of concern and my trust in authority continued throughout my life. I've always been able to hold up well under adversity and sometimes even step it up a notch when faced with catastrophe. I don't rattle easily, and I think that when I was hit with the incredibly severe form of Guillain-Barré Syndrome, this ability to cope probably did as much as any healing processes to keep me alive.

CHAPTER TEN

SLOW MOTION

When faced with dangerous situations, people react in different ways. Some will totally freeze up. Some will run away. Some will make terrible decisions, which often intensify a situation. Some will break down in tears. I've seen them all occur during the many serious, and sometimes dangerous, circumstances in which I've found myself.

It's been my experience, when faced with a serious or potentially dangerous or violent circumstance, that I do the complete opposite. My mind seems to go into a slow-motion mode rather than intensify. It's as if my vision becomes a camera that zooms in on the root of the problem, and I start evaluating the steps I should take to solve the problem. To what stage has the situation grown? What can I do to deescalate the problem? Is the environment safe? Is anyone immediately available to help me and, if not, is there anyone in the general area who could help? How can I contact others for help? What are the consequences should this situation get out of hand? How much time do I have?

There are a million things to consider in times like these, and a tremendous number of them run through my mind when I'm faced with an urgent situation. But as I begin evaluating all these things, I also begin to act as I see fit, continuing to process next steps. That's just the way I'm wired and I feel that this makeup helped me survive as I faced the possibility of a terrible outcome, possibly even death, during my ordeal with Guillain-Barré.

I've been asked the same question hundreds of times when I describe the day the condition hit me. That question is, "Weren't you scared? You had to be terrified!"

My response is always the same. "No, I wasn't scared. I had confidence in the fact that I was in a hospital and I knew they would fix me." I didn't fall apart. I didn't break down and imagine the worst-case scenario. I didn't feel sorry for myself. I didn't freak out. I kept my shit together and my mind started evaluating everything. I was trying to come up with a solution. I fell back on what I'd learned regarding situations of this nature.

Yes, I was concerned. I was more concerned than I had probably ever been in my life; but I had the experience of many tough situations to fall back on. And that insurance, my friends, became more valuable than anything Blue Cross Blue Shield ever provided.

In 1984 or '85, we were playing a club in Norfolk, Virginia, where we worked on a regular basis. One night, we had just finished our last set and the lights had come up. It was a normal night; people were finishing up their last drinks, saying goodbye to each other, and eventually working their way toward the door. For the band and road crew, our duties varied at this point based on whether we were playing another night in the same place or tearing down, packing up, and heading to another city. On this particular evening, we had the luxury of playing another night, so all we had to do was get the guitars cleaned and put away, and cover up the rest of the instruments. As for my equipment, it meant taking down the vocal mics, covering my sound board and associated outboard gear, and packing up the T-shirts and caps I hadn't sold to take them back to the hotel with me. I was in the process of covering the board with a big packing quilt that I carried for this purpose. Jonna was there and she was helping me out with this ritual.

Suddenly, I heard angry yelling near the entrance of the club. I snapped my head around to see about six people standing there. The main one yelling was the night manager, Paul. Paul was filling in for Allen, the regular manager.

As a road manager, at the venues we played I usually dealt with the promoter or, in the case of smaller venues such as this one, the night manager. So, I knew Paul well from past jobs. Paul was a great guy who knew his job, but he also had a short fuse and took no shit at all. Evidently, someone in this group of people had tried to give Paul some shit and his fuse had quickly been lit.

I walked toward them while Paul was ordering some guy to get out. The guy, whom I'd never seen before, flatly told Paul that he'd leave when he got good and ready to do so. The guy in question was a pretty good-sized individual who looked to be in his early twenties. I hadn't noticed any problems all night and to this day I have no idea what precipitated this exchange.

Paul again loudly told the guy to hit the road and the man again refused so Paul hollered, "We'll see about that!" He turned and walked in the opposite direction.

I asked the fellow what the deal was, and he told me he wasn't going to be talked to that way. As soon as he said that, here came Paul hurrying back. Again, Paul ordered the guy to get out and again the guy said something to the effect of, "Make me."

At this point Paul pulled a pistol out of his pocket and pointed it right at the guy's face from a distance of about four feet. Point-blank range. Again, Paul told him to get out, but this time also stated, "Or I'll kill you!"

I remember thinking, *Dan, you gotta do something or this is going to get real bad, real quick.* So, I stepped in between the fellow, who was about to be renamed "the victim," and the pistol that Paul was about to fire.

I looked at Paul and said, "Paul, just lay the gun down, and I'll get rid of this guy, and the night will be over."

Paul looked at me for a few seconds. No one spoke a word. Finally, Paul laid the gun on a nearby table. Jonna, who had made her way to the scene, happened to be standing right beside the table. We made instant eye contact and I nodded toward the gun. Without hesitation, she picked it up and took off toward the kitchen behind the bar.

I turned to the guy in question and calmly told him, "It's all over, just get on your way, and this night will be over, and we can all live to see another day." He didn't utter another word as he turned and walked out the door. I never saw him again. Sometimes you just gotta do what you gotta do.

CHAPTER ELEVEN

DREAMS AND HALLUCINATIONS

During my six-month hospital stay, I was administered medications liberally. I wanted to know how much medication was given to me, either orally or through an IV. (Then again, maybe it's better that I never know. If someone were to make me aware of the exact amount and the types, it could very well put me into cardiac arrest—and then we'd have a new problem.)

When I was conscious again and found myself housed at St. Joseph's, I received an unexpected gift from all these medications—a string of hallucinations and the most vivid dreams I've ever had. Some were entertaining. Some were interesting. Some were quite comical, and some were scary—downright terrifying, to be honest. The dreams seemed to come every time I went to sleep, which was often. Over the first three weeks, I was probably asleep as many, if not more, hours than I was awake.

This was good and necessary so my body could start repairing itself, but at the same time it was bad when the more unsettling dreams decided to show up.

One of the more troubling dreams centered around my being connected to a ventilator. With my awareness that this machine's operation was necessary for my life support, I had a subconscious fear that it would fail and I would suffocate. This was nearly impossible, as it had an alarm that activated whenever the least thing went wrong, and this alarm was incredibly loud. It did legitimately sound off a few times for whatever reason; and when it did, nurses would come flying into my room at breakneck speed to correct the problem, which was always minor. This increased my confidence in the ventilator and subsequently put my mind at ease, at least when I was awake. I was not always awake.

While sleeping, I would think I was gasping for air. The same nurse was always in this nightmare, even though it took place under many different circumstances. Sometimes we were in my room. Sometimes we were in a different room. Sometimes we were in a different area of the hospital, and sometimes we weren't even in the hospital. I don't know to this day if this nurse was one of my regular caregivers or if she was someone my sleeping mind had conjured up on its own. It seemed that she was someone I knew from the street, from my hometown even. I never knew her name; but it wouldn't have done me any good to know it because I was unable to speak because of that damned—no, blessed—ventilator.

No matter the setting of my dream, the machine would malfunction and I would have trouble breathing. For some reason in these dreams, I was able to move. In real life I couldn't walk or even leave my bed for that matter, but I could move in my dreams. I'd begin waving my arms or hitting the side of the mattress, anything to get her attention. Sometimes my dream-world caregiver would notice me, but other times she'd be oblivious.

A common occurrence in this dream was for my nurse to acknowledge my signals of distress but to seemingly dismiss them. She would say, "I see you, but you'll have to wait. I'm doing something else right now. You'll be alright." These dreams were the hardest to get through. She knew I was in trouble, but she wasn't willing to help me right then. She showed no emotion, which exasperated me. I was scared to death, and she could have put my mind at rest by physically attending to me—and she knew it—but she was going to do it in her own sweet time.

As terrifying as these nightmares were, they always ended well. She'd always get over to me after what seemed like an eternity to fix whatever the problem was, and I'd be able to breathe normally again and then slowly drift off to sleep.

Not all my dreams were frightening. Another one, which came up almost every night for several nights, was not only interesting but also eventually became humorous. In these dreams I imagined that I wasn't a patient. I believed that I was an employee and my job was to leave the hospital every day at the end of my shift to accompany one or more of the nurses home. Male nurses some days. Female nurses other days. Some nights we'd just go to a house and spend time together, doing what anyone else would do: have dinner, watch TV, read a book, then go to bed. The next morning whoever had been with me would somehow get me back to the hospital in time to start my shift as an employee again.

During these illusory experiences, I would have regained not only the ability to move—even though I still couldn't get out of the bed—but also the ability speak with no problem; and the ventilator would have magically disappeared. I would, in fact, have long conversations with whomever my companion was for the night. This was quite liberating, to say the least.

I have ideas as to the significance of this type of experience but am far from schooled in evaluating such things, so I won't attempt an explanation. I also don't have an explanation for the most common hallucination I experienced.

Even though the hallucinations were many and varied, one happened pretty much daily. It occurred when I was fully awake and acutely aware of everything going on around me. It consisted of my seeing a groundhog-like creature appear in a corner along one edge of the ceiling and scurry across that edge of ceiling, disappearing down behind the door that opened into my room. I witnessed this whether anyone else was present or not. At first it was a little unsettling, but as the frequency of visits from my little furry friend increased, I was almost glad to see him at times. He let me know I was awake and alive.

One day, just before I was transferred to the rehab facility, a male nurse came into my room and was talking to me when he saw my eyes shift toward the ceiling and scan from the corner to the door. He asked what I was looking at, and I just smiled and replied, "Man, you really wouldn't understand."

CHAPTER TWELVE

NEW YEAR'S EVE

Back in the late '80s, as I'm sure is still the case today, the New Year's Eve job was the most profitable of the year for any act. This was because almost any venue you played could charge a higher ticket fee for that night based on the extra amenities they would provide like free champagne at midnight, free snacks, fireworks, and just an overall New Year's Eve party experience. We had booked the job in Jacksonville, North Carolina, at a club called PJ's. Jacksonville is home to Camp Lejeune, one of the largest Marine Corps bases in the United States. We always did well in military towns since the young guys in the military, for the most part, had a mindset that went right along with our style of music, hard rock. We had played PJ's several times before and always drew a big crowd. This was particularly appealing to me because I owned all our merchandising rights, and military guys were always willing customers for T-shirts, caps, and the rest. I even had special shirts printed for this night with "New Year's Eve 1985, Jacksonville, North Carolina" printed on the back. I ordered five dozen of these shirts and, as it turned out that night, we had a capacity crowd of 1500. I sold everything I had. Our contract for that night was the largest we'd ever signed. It wasn't the events of that night so much as it was those that occurred the day before that I'll forever remember.

We always tried our best to take off Christmas and the few days around it in order to provide some home time for the guys in the band and the road crew. That year was no exception. We'd just finished a six-week schedule that had taken us mostly to the Deep South. We finished up on December 23rd in Pascagoula, Mississippi. As soon as the trailer was loaded, I fired up that old International tractor trailer and headed home to Virginia Beach with a couple of guys from the crew whom I dropped off along the way. I was especially looking forward to getting back home, as I had gone on a high-protein, low-carb diet on this trip and succeeded in dropping forty pounds—so I was excited to see Jonna's reaction to my weight loss.

The holiday went well, and before I knew it, it was time to hit the road again. I left for Jacksonville on December 30th. It was a four-hour drive down Highway 17, which was predominately a two-lane road running across the Virginia/North Carolina state line. A beautiful drive, mostly through rolling, wooded farmland. It was a trip that I'd made many times.

On the way down, I had as my traveling companions Brian Watts, our stage manager, and Scott Banevich, who went on to fame as the bass player for the Edwin McCain band in the late '90s and early 2000s when McCain gained national exposure with the release of back-to-back albums that both went platinum. We left out early that morning, about 10:00 AM. Well, that was early for us, anyway. Rock 'n' rollers weren't big on getting up early.

A little over an hour into our trip, I began to sense something was wrong with the truck's engine. It just didn't seem to have the power that it normally did. I'd checked the oil level just the day before, as that engine had always used oil; and we'd had the oil pump replaced a few months before. It had been running just fine, but on this day something wasn't right. It felt weak. Suddenly it lost power and the engine nearly shut down. I was on one of those two-lane stretches of asphalt that ran through farmland, so I started looking for any place to pull off immediately. Luckily, I spotted a long, wide spot on the shoulder ahead, so I mashed in the clutch and let it coast to a stop at the side of the road. I tried to restart it, but the engine wouldn't turn over. I didn't know it at the time, but this would be the last time I'd ever drive that old truck. Evidently, the oil pump had decided to expire again, and this time it took out the entire bottom end of the engine. It wasn't worth the money it was going to take to repair it. Turns out that the death of the

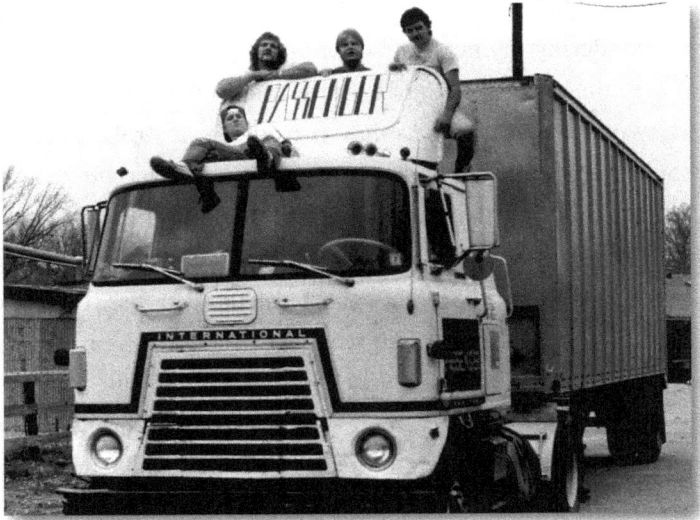

Road crew for Passenger, somewhere on the East Coast, circa 1983

tractor trailer was a precursor to the death of the band. This would prove to be our last New Year's Eve performance and the band would break up six months later. I really hated to see that ride go. We'd always taken pride in having a tractor trailer. I knew of only one other bar band in the Carolinas who had one; and believe me, back in the '80s, before the legal drinking age changed, there were a lot of bar bands. That other band was called Sidewinder. They were based in eastern North Carolina and had won for thirteen consecutive weeks on *Star Search*, a predecessor to TV shows like *American Idol*, which would come along many years later. We played the same circuit.

That experience of *slow-down-and-evaluate-the-situation-so-you-can-fix-it-expediently* thing took over my mind. First, I realized that we were in the middle of nowhere, so I would have to find a way to contact someone for help. This was long before cell phones, so my immediate thought was to flag someone down and get a ride to a pay phone—not an attractive option because I'd have to hitch a ride back to the truck after the phone call. Pondering my next move, I noticed a gravel driveway just off the other side of the road. At the end of the driveway sat an old, two-story farmhouse. Man, it would be a stroke of luck if people were home and had a phone that they'd let me use.

I told the guys that I'd walk up to the farmhouse and see if they had a phone. I put on the coat that I'd just received as a Christmas gift and started my short trek to the house. I knocked on the door. Shortly, an older woman opened the door. She was probably in her seventies, and I introduced myself. I told her the truth: "I'm driving a tractor trailer and it's broken down on the side of the road right there." I pointed to it. I asked her if she had a phone I could use. Her husband stepped into our conversation, and I reiterated my request. They both agreed.

They seemed friendly enough, and I was grateful they were home and were willing to let a stranger come in and use their phone.

I walked into a classic old Southern farmhouse kitchen. I smelled food cooking. I couldn't identify exactly what it was, but it made me feel at home. It was discernibly different from all the restaurants where I'd been eating for several years. I felt comfortable right away. My reception was different from what I'd expected.

Their phone hung on the wall at the edge of the kitchen; and I used it to call our drummer, who owned 50 percent of the band and was the only one of us who knew much about mechanics. In fact, after leaving the band, he met and married a girl whose family was in the trucking business, and together they still manage that same successful company.

He told me he'd get in touch with the club owner in Jacksonville, explain our plight, and inquire about helping us out. After a short time, he called back to tell me the club owner was sending another tractor to pull ours back to Jacksonville so we could save the job. He was a very nice guy and, let's face it, this job was just as important to him as it was to us. It was going to be several hours before the other truck would arrive, so it looked as if Brian, Scott, and I would have a lengthy wait on our hands.

***

There's a difference between being in a band and being in a road band. Most bands today just play sporadically or on the weekends. The band members have day jobs or some other way to support their music lifestyle. This was not the case in a true road band. Playing in front of an audience was our profession. We lived it day in and day out. This profession and accompanying lifestyle do not exist today—or if it does, it exists on a much smaller scale. Back in the '80s, many bands used this arrangement as their livelihood. Again, this was before the drinking age increased from eighteen to twenty-one, and that changed things for everyone. I truly think the change in the legal drinking age contributed to the downfall in the quality of music that's presented to the consumer today. Fans will never have the opportunity to choose entertainment as it was back then. The consumer today is at the mercy of the record companies. Whatever is shoved down your throat is what you'll have to either accept or reject. It wasn't always that way. Back then, public perception of a live concert they heard the night before in a local club could ultimately influence the future of that act.

I've often heard the analogy that being in a band is like being married to the other members of the band. This is not true. If you're married to someone, you'll usually be around them for a lot of hours each day—but not all the hours in the day. Job constraints or other obligations will remove you from that spouse on almost a daily basis. In a road band this is not the case. You are around each other constantly. Twenty-four hours a day. Every day. Life is much more concentrated. You learn to be acutely aware of the other members' habits, likes, and dislikes. It might even be more personal than being married. It evolves into a lifestyle that you don't even realize is transpiring. The routine of being in a normal family atmosphere erodes, whether you want it to or not. You adapt to life on the road—or you get out.

What happened that day back in 1985 brought Brian and Scott and me back into that family atmosphere, if only for a few hours. That old couple in the farmhouse took us in as if we were family, and it's a memory we'll always treasure.

When I asked if my friends waiting in the truck could come in and wait until we got a solution to our plight (or at least further instructions from our other band members), they didn't hesitate to invite us in. The wife said she was surprised that I hadn't already asked them to come inside their house, as it was a cold December day; and since the truck wasn't running, they had no heat.

Even with this overwhelming exhibition of hospitality, I was still a bit hesitant when it came to ask them to join us. I always had a knack for being able to make people feel comfortable, even if we had just met. Brian and Scott were both very amiable individuals; but even though I had long hair at the time, I didn't know how our hosts would respond to a couple more long-haired rock 'n' rollers coming into their home.

At any rate, I walked out to the truck, explained the situation and our options, and walked back to the house with my friends in tow. What happened next is the most delightful part of this memory. The couple didn't gasp. They didn't look uncertain. They didn't hesitate in any way. They invited my friends in just as they had invited me.

We spent the next few hours sharing stories. We learned as much or more about them as they learned about us. Before dinner, we went into their living room where a twenty-five-inch TV was on, and the husband asked what we'd like to watch. I, never being at a loss to decide, suggested that we watch the NFL playoffs, as this was a Sunday and the conference championships were on. No hesitation. He welcomed me to get up and change the channel myself. Yep, there were few remote-controlled TVs back in those days. We sat there watching the game, and before long the wife came in and announced that supper was almost ready. She asked us to help ourselves, which we did—eagerly. Fried chicken, mashed potatoes and gravy, green beans, and everything else you would imagine coming out of a classic country kitchen. We sat there with our plates on our laps, as there wasn't enough space around their small dining room table for us all, and we thoroughly enjoyed our meal and each other's company. I didn't want the experience to end. I was loving it. For a fleeting moment, all three of us were removed from our everyday band experience and transported back into the family time that we didn't even realize we had been missing.

After dark another truck did appear, along with a car; the trailer was hooked up for its final trip to Jacksonville. Brian and Scott rode in the car, but I—as a faithful warrior—rode with the truck driver up in the cab. Before leaving, I offered to pay our gracious hosts for the meal and their hospitality, but as has always been the case in the South, they would have no part of it. Instead, they thanked us for giving them a New Year's experience they would always remember.

I fully intended to return to their old farmhouse one day and formally show my gratitude for a day we'd always remember as well; but as things turned out, I never had the opportunity. To this day I can still picture that house at the end of the gravel driveway after knowing our faithful tractor trailer had called it quits—and hoping beyond hope that the occupants of that house would help us out. Not being able to convey that message has always been one of my greatest regrets. Maybe it was intended to turn out that way.

CHAPTER THIRTEEN

FRIENDSHIP WITH MY CAREGIVERS

Anytime you're around the same group of people for an extended period, you tend to develop a personal relationship with them. Sometimes good relationships. Sometimes bad. This is especially true in a work or school environment. Think about how often you hear of two co-workers who become romantically involved. Sometimes it even leads to marriage. You walk off into the sunset with the guy or girl of your dreams and live happily ever after.

This can also work in the reverse. Just think about all the times you've heard of a marriage ruined due to a relationship that developed in a work environment. Think of all the times, especially today, that you hear of a disgruntled co-worker or student walking into a workplace or school and opening fire, killing everybody in range.

The story doesn't always have a fairy tale ending. Sometimes it ends in disaster. But both have one thing in common—they originated in an environment which placed the participants in close proximity to each other on a recurring basis. It's human nature. When you're regularly face to face with the same people, relationships are bound to develop.

I've learned that the same is true in a hospital environment. The only difference is that there isn't one but two groups of people. It's not only the employees intermingling every day, the patients also come into the picture if they're admitted for a sufficient period. I guess I can compare this situation to what occurs in a prison environment, where the inmates are cast into a role like that of a patient. In a hospital it's the duty of the staff to provide for the well-being of the patients. The same is true in prison. It's the duty of the staff to provide for the well-being of the inmates. Sometimes this evolves into a romantic relationship, and sometimes it goes south. I can't tell you how many times over the years I saw fellow staff members get familiar with inmates, and I also saw staff get physically assaulted by inmates who couldn't take another day of having to listen to "that son of a bitch" who "disrespected" them on a daily basis.

Luckily, in all my months of hospital confinement, no relationship that I developed turned sour. There were really good people taking care of me, and (with the exception of only one therapist) I truly believe everyone had my health and best interest at heart. In any good relationship, you'll have something in common with the other person. More with some. Less with others. But you're still in a personal relationship, and hopefully both participants will seek to learn more about the other and enjoy being around them.

All my life I've found myself in day-to-day contact with others, no matter what my job or responsibilities were at the time. There was always the normal conversation and banter that I now realize is essential to my mindset. I needed that and thrived on it. In the hospital, unable to speak, I didn't have it. I could only observe others and listen to their words. I couldn't respond, and I needed that connection in the worst way. Communication would be another way for me to return to normal. I hungered for the opportunity to converse with others, and when it finally did arise, I was elated! The day I was removed from the ventilator, I was suddenly empowered with the ability to speak again and the opportunity to form relationships. This was tremendous! I had become very close to these caregivers—at least in my mind—and I wanted so much to finally give back to them what they had given to me: my time and attention in the form of a few words out of my mouth.

All animals can communicate with one another. Humans are no different. Even those who are mute learn sign language to get their thoughts across. This ability had been taken away from me except for shaking or nodding my head until I started to point at letters on a page or board. It was a very lonely feeling. I could absorb information, thoughts, and feelings, but couldn't respond to them. This was a tremendous hindrance in fostering a relationship. It was another thing I'd never thought of. I had to adapt and overcome, so I just tried to keep my mind strong and my outlook positive until the day I could verbally communicate again—and when that day came, I made the most of it.

As time has passed, I've had the opportunity to speak with many of the former caregivers I was around every day. One thing that's been consistent in their evaluation of my ability to speak again is that they loved finally hearing my voice but couldn't get me to "shut the hell up!" I was also told this by my visitors. Well so be it; I had a lot of catching up to do.

I really did want to get closer to those who took care of me, and I've always found that a good way to start a conversation is to find a point of mutual interest. I came up with an icebreaker question so I could get a reaction and the chance to increase interest. I hoped it would lead further, to more personal topics, which is the best way to start a true relationship. I finally came up with that one-size-fits-all icebreaker. I tried it and it worked.

Asheville is the largest city west of Charlotte in North Carolina. It's a beautiful, progressive tourist destination, as well as a great place to live. Asheville also has, by far, the highest cost of living around, possibly higher than any other city in the state. It's where all three hospitals I was housed in are located. With that in mind, the icebreaker I asked nearly every person who walked through my door was, "Do you live in Asheville?" Almost 90 percent answered no, then proceeded to share where they did live. I knew it would turn out that way. I'd then respond with something to the effect of, "Yeah, I would love to live in Asheville, but I can't afford it." It always led to a discussion of how ridiculous the housing market in Asheville was. It was just a common, ordinary topic, but one that anyone could relate to and thus, give me my chance to make our conversation more personal. That's the way an icebreaker ought to work. Beats the heck out of, "Nice weather we're having, huh?"

Through my adult life, I've discovered that I have the power of understanding and inclusion during a conversation that develops a relationship. I don't mean this facetiously. I think by simply talking to people, you can accomplish what talking is designed for. You find out what they're interested in or concerned about, and they in turn discover the same things about you. This is why I believe we have the ability to communicate. And I'm not referring to modern day communication such as texting or social media. Those are rudimentary. Too impersonal. Open, honest communication is the key to solving a lot of problems. I often used to teach that, within the prison environment, physical intimidation means nothing, even though new hires often thought so. Talking face-to-face still accomplishes more than any computer-supported sharing of thoughts that exists today. I had a lot of health problems to solve and I knew that these were exactly the people who could help me solve them. Hell, they were the only people who could help me and at last I had an avenue to connect more directly and personally with them. Finally, I could speak whenever I wanted to, if even I was doing so lying on my back.

***

Nearly all the staff who cared for me were nice people. When I gained the ability to converse, a lot of them morphed from just being nice people to being friends of mine. Before I could speak, I could see that they were genuinely happy to see me when they came by to check on me, but that enjoyment had noticeably intensified. It was no longer a matter of just asking me how I was doing and looking down to acknowledge a head nod. They could expect me to say that I was doing well or that I was having problems—I have no difficulty telling someone if I'm having problems.

The greeting I hate more than any other is, "Hi, how are you doing today?" It serves no purpose. Even if the guy who was asked that question had just had both legs severed below the knee in a chainsaw accident, he would invariably reply, "Fine, how are you?" Total waste of time.

Whenever I'm greeted in that way, I almost never respond as expected. Even if I'm doing fine, I'll usually say something to the effect of, "Could be worse." That's one of my favorites. If nothing else it makes the person who greeted me stop for a moment and consider that, yes, it could indeed be worse, it means I got her brain active for just a moment and maybe, just maybe, she'll choose to engage a little better sometime.

As I got to know the staff better, I learned more about their favorite interests. There was one first-shift male CNA. I found he had a great interest in sports, as did I. During football season, we spent a lot of time talking about college and pro football. Finally our relationship evolved to the point that, if there were games that interested him on TV the days he was working, he'd stop by my room every chance he got, and the first thing out of his mouth wasn't, "How are you doing?" It was more like, "How are the Panthers doing?" This was fine with me. Believe me, I would have told him if I was having any problems, and it gave him a little break from his busy duties to get away for a couple of minutes.

As a matter of fact, as time went on, a lot of the staff at St. Joseph's learned that 404 was somewhere they could escape to for a couple of minutes and at the same time have a leisurely conversation with a guy who wanted to listen to them and hear what they had to say. I had no problem whatsoever with that. When you've been essentially alone inside yourself for as long as I was, you welcome the interaction.

Before this experience, I never gave much thought to what hospital staff members had to deal with daily. I had worked many jobs in which I had to deal with the public, and I took it for granted that it was pretty much the same everywhere. I was wrong. I observed many patients who were delusional. Hell, I was delusional from time to time. The patients I'm talking about here were not only delusional—some were downright violent. Several times during my stay a patient had to be physically restrained. I didn't get to witness these instances, but I overheard them happening. Other patients felt they were more privileged than anyone else in the joint; they came across as total assholes. I guess you get them in any business.

But the ones who must have been the most difficult were those who were either terminally ill or close to it; I guess I was one of them for a time. Imagine how difficult it must be in any profession to deal with people who are most certainly going to die while in your care. The emotional strain is something I don't believe I could endure for very long. People in this line of work do deal with this, sometimes during every shift. I believe when they encounter a patient like me, one who hasn't given up and is someone they can talk easily with during their shift, they must surely appreciate that fact.

A memorable interaction with a staff member occurred one day when I tried to talk a nurse into helping me get up on my feet so I could show him I could walk on my own. This was a day when either some of my medication must have been mistakenly increased. Or I was having one of my hallucinations. This guy was the head nurse on one of the first-shift rotations. He came into my room to check on me. For some reason I had it in my mind that I had magically regained the ability to walk on my own two feet after being flat on my back for over three months. I believed it with all my heart or at least that's what I told him. It must have come to me in an epiphany. Or a dream. This nurse and I had developed a pretty good relationship, and he remembered seeing me working out at the YMCA in Marion before I got sick. He and his wife used to work out in the evening about the same time I did. After being reminded of this, I also recognized him; so I figured if anyone would be open to my request for assistance to get up and walk, it would be him. I threw the notion out there and he brushed me off at first, but I persisted. On this day I had convinced myself that I could get up and go for a walk about the place. He finally told me that I had been paralyzed long enough to almost completely atrophy my muscles, and it would be medically impossible for me to snap back, just like that. I listened to what he had to say, but I wouldn't shut up—so he finally told me that he'd make a deal with me. He said that if I could just sit up on the side of the bed, he would then help me to my feet and happily accompany me on a walk to wherever I chose to go.

This sounded reasonable, so I decided to take him up on it and told him, "Just watch me."

Even though I tried with all the might I could muster, I was unsuccessful even to sit up. I could barely get one shoulder started in the right direction, so I finally accepted his explanation as fact and drifted off to sleep. I'm sure he walked around the rest of the day with a little smile on his face; but as I look back, he handled the situation very professionally. He listened to what I said. He explained my actual situation to me. He even gave me an option to show him I had the ability to earn his help by showing him that I could make a physical effort. What he did not do was ignore me, laugh at me, or make derogatory comments to me, which would have been easy for him to do. The staff had to encounter this type of behavior every time they punched in, and my hat's off to them for being able to take it. Working with human beings can be taxing when they're healthy. I can't imagine doing it with those who were anything but.

***

Another staff member who sticks out in my mind was a lead nurse on the night shift. Her name was Lindsey, and we hit it off immediately. She had a great personality—and it sure didn't hurt that she was drop-dead gorgeous. The first time I saw her I remember thinking, *If I was just thirty years younger...* But I wasn't. So, again, I was just looking to make a friend. We did become friends and we stay in contact to this day. I recall a day after I was able to speak once more, when she came into my room at about 4:00 a.m. to give me my medication. On this morning, I noticed that she had her hair down instead of pinned up. Most of the nurses wore their hair up most of the time, as I'm sure it was much quicker and easier to deal with—not to mention keeping it out of the way while they were working. Anyway, for some reason seeing her with her hair draped over her shoulders and down her back hit me as being especially beautiful. Never being one who had a hard time expressing myself, I told her so. Before I even thought about what I was saying, I said, "Lindsey, you've got beautiful hair. You should wear it down more often."

The next two nights I was tickled to see my second-shift lead nurse come in with her hair flowing down her back. I couldn't help thinking, just for an instant, *Dan, you've still got it.* When I brought this up to her a couple years later, she said that she remembered me making that statement and how it had made her night. I'll never forget that.

A young lady by the name of Charlotte was assigned as my respiratory therapist. She primarily also worked night shifts with Lindsey. The thing that hit me about Charlotte was the fact that she bore a striking resemblance to a girl I had worked with in my department store retail days years before. The first time she walked into my room I actually thought it was my old friend and each time I see her to this day that's the first thing that pops into my mind.

Having to depend on a ventilator for every breath of life I took at that time made Charlotte a particularly important participant in my adventure. I couldn't deny the importance that the ventilator played in my day-to-day existence. It literally meant the difference between life and death. Therefore, I loved that apparatus.

It was adjusted to alarm if the least thing did not quite meet the specifications it was programmed to detect and, let me tell you, it detected these slight abnormalities in an instant. That damn thing would sound an alarm at the drop of a hat, and it wasn't a subdued alarm, it was just what the word is meant to imply, it was an ALARM. Therefore, I hated that apparatus. Staff members were constantly in and out, checking each time it sounded off. I'm sure it was somewhat annoying to them, but they were of course used to it because they had to deal with it every day. It was just part of the job. But it drove me crazy and there wasn't a thing I could do about it except lie there and wait for someone to come in and reset it. However, like everything else in life, if you experience anything long enough, you tend to get used to it and the ventilator alarm was no different. Slowly, the alarms fell farther into the recesses of my mind.

The number one thing I will always remember about Charlotte though was when she would bring in this portable hand-held vibrator device. She would press it against my chest and move it around in an effort to keep the phlegm inside my lungs loosened up to make it easier to suction out. Actually, a very important piece of equipment. To me it was more than this, however. I have been fortunate enough to have received professional massages on more than one occasion as well as impromptu massages from time to time when I found myself in the right place at the right time, if you know what I mean, and I truly believe that a good massage it one of life's greatest pleasures. Even though I wasn't able to express it early on, I can assure you that my personality and attitude brightened immensely each time I saw Charlotte walk through my door with the little chest vibrator massager thing in hand. I can somewhat equate it to how a puppy acts when its owner comes through the door of the house after a hard day's work. It is overjoyed to see its master finally get home and expresses this joy by running around, barking, and incessantly wagging its tail. Well I couldn't run around, bark, much less wag my tail, but I sure wanted to every time I saw Charlotte walk in carrying that chest massage pleasure machine. I knew that things were about to get better if only for a few minutes, but they were a few minutes that were enjoyed immensely and will I always treasure.

I guess one of the most special moments with the folks operating the LTAC floor came on Christmas Day. My dear friend Tonya, who could easily be the subject of an entire chapter, was planning to spend Christmas Day with me, and I had proudly shared this fact with anyone who was close enough to hear my voice.

I'd spoken with most of my caregivers about how they liked to enjoy the holiday. Most of them had special, family-oriented activities during Christmastime. Most were the things you would expect: dinner with the family, wrapping presents, singing carols, drinking eggnog. They'd always ask me if I had anything special that I liked to do, and I told them about a movie made back when I was a kid, *The Homecoming: A Christmas Story*, which launched the highly successful TV series, *The Waltons*. It was a tradition in our house to get together and watch *The Homecoming* each year. When my parents got their first VCR, this was one of the first recordings I ever made for them. I also made a copy for myself, and I related to the nurses that I'd saved that tape and still watched it each Yuletide; and if I hadn't been in the hospital, I'd have been watching it again. I'd always get the obligatory "Ahhhs" when I relayed this story, and they'd follow it up with an offer to make it as nice as they could for me.

Well, Christmas Day finally arrived and, sure enough, right around lunchtime my beautiful Tonya walked in. We hugged, smiled, and laughed a lot—and probably didn't shut up for more than a couple of seconds for the first half hour. Tonya and I never had a problem with communication. Each time we got together, whether it had been three months since we had seen each other or three minutes, we were never at a loss for something to talk about.

Finally, in walked the first-shift head nurse Alisha. You remember her from the Coca-Cola/swallow-test story. Alisha handed me a small package. I was completely humbled but overjoyed at the same time. Suddenly, I was a little kid on Christmas morning, getting ready to unwrap my first present. I thanked her and, removing the wrapping paper, what do you think I found inside? That's right, ladies and gentlemen, a DVD of *The Homecoming*. I nearly started crying right there, and I think I did have to wipe away a couple of little tears anyway. I was so touched that this woman, not only my nurse but my friend, took the time to make one of her patients' Christmas wishes come true. I was truly touched.

Right at that very moment, in walked Omar, the second-shift lead nurse who worked the rotation opposite from Lindsey. I was surprised to see him, and I asked what he was doing there at this time of day.

He said, "Well, I brought something for you," and pulled out a wrapped package from behind his back. I unwrapped it and what do you think it was? We have a winner! Another DVD of *The Homecoming*. I nearly jumped out of the bed and hugged him, but as you remember, I wasn't quite at that point yet. Alisha and Omar said they hadn't talked to each other about my mentioning the movie. They had each just taken it upon themselves, independently, to do something for an old guy who was spending Christmas in the hospital.

Tonya and I sat back and relaxed in room 404 to watch my favorite Christmas movie. My heart was smiling, even if my face couldn't show it. After Alisha and Omar left the room, Tonya looked at me and said, "Well, it looks like you've made a couple of friends."

I happily replied, "Yes, I have."

CHAPTER FOURTEEN

TOUGH TIMES IN OUR LIVES

We all encounter adversity. Some more than others. Some people experience so much hardship that it seems as if they have a dark cloud hanging over them from the day they are born. More often, however, people have major disasters come upon them randomly and only occasionally. The effects of these episodes on one's security and well-being can be wide ranging. Some people drown in hardships, never to return fully to life. Most of the time, an individual goes through a tough time, struggles through it, and somehow surfaces again in the end.

The general make-up of the individual and the circumstances surrounding these disasters determine if a fellow will weather the storm—or if it will destroy, severely alter, adversely effect, or in the most severe cases, end his life. This is where suicide enters the picture—an extreme solution to this suffering.

Many look at people who choose to take their own lives as not just troubled and desperate, but also as selfish. Many times I've heard someone say something like, "How could he have been so selfish as to leave his family and friends behind to deal with life's problems on their own?" It may look this way from the outside, and you may think that this is the politically correct thing to say; but until you've had the things going on inside your mind that the suicide victim had going on in his, I don't understand how someone could respond with such harsh judgment.

People take their own lives for an array of reasons. Unrequited romantic relationships, money problems, severe embarrassment, bullying, medical issues, pain . . . the list goes on and on. I'm not saying that taking your own life is the right thing to do, but I am saying that you never know how you'll react to a debilitating situation until you face it.

I've been through several severe and traumatizing incidents during my life, and none was more traumatizing than my battle with Guillain-Barré Syndrome. It was devastating to go from completely healthy to completely paralyzed in a twenty-four-hour period. And then to be told two weeks later that the only known treatments aren't working . . . and the future looks bad enough to put me into a sedated state . . . and we'll just hope for the best. It was stunning.

I did have a couple of things going for me though. The first is my general mental makeup in dealing with adversity. Another was that I hadn't been told my condition was terminal. The most obvious was that I was completely paralyzed. Hell, I couldn't have done anything drastic even if I had wanted to. Lastly, by the time I wasn't sedated any longer, the worst had passed, and it was up to me how quickly, or if, I would recover and to what degree.

The major thing I want to accomplish in writing this book is simple. I want to give encouragement to you who are going through a devastating time—to give you hope that there's a reason to keep trying to improve. Somehow you must gather yourself, determine a plan of action, and then put everything you've got into accomplishing your goal. It may be tough, but it is possible.

I've seen the following scenario play out with many people. Tragedy occurs. They're completely devastated. The mental outlook is bleak. The mountain seems too high to climb, and they wonder if it's even worth climbing.

I can assure you that the answer to that last question is an unequivocal, loud YES! I've never seen even one of these people improve their physical or mental well-being by just sitting around feeling sorry for themselves. That attitude only causes the entire situation to deteriorate. If you think your life is bad now, give it a few months or years of mourning the situation, and you'll see just how bad it can get. You can ignore it as best you can, but it's always going to be right there in your mind, even if you shove it as far back as you can.

If you'll take the other approach and put forth your honest best effort, I can almost guarantee that your life will improve, and you'll probably improve the lives of those around you along the way.

Remember how I explained the necessity of learning how to lose and coming back from it and handling it—because life is going to deal you some bad hands along the way? Well, that's the crux of this book. You win a few. You lose a few. But there's always another game to play.

CHAPTER FIFTEEN

LAST DAYS AT ST. JOSEPH'S

Well, the rough days in the LTAC at St. Joseph's Hospital seemed to be coming to an end. With a therapist's help, I was gaining a little more movement each day. I saw significant progress. Until this point, the only staff working with me were from a purely medical point of view. Not that therapists aren't members of the medical treatment community. They certainly are; but to me, they're more closely related to physical fitness, an area that I understood. I didn't know a lot about monitoring one's internal organs or evaluating the interaction of the immune system with the nervous system, but I did know quite a bit about the human muscular system and its relationship to the skeletal structure. During my long involvement in athletics, I had to rebound from various injuries, so I had a rough idea of what I'd be facing in therapy. I'd never encountered anything as complex as this, but I was more than willing to get on with it. However, during my first stages of physical rehabilitation, I ran across the only staff member that I really had a problem with during my entire six-month hospital stay.

He was a male physical therapist in his mid-fifties. He walked with an air of purpose, but at the same time seemed to be consumed only with the words coming out of his own mouth, not processing what was said to him. He appeared to think he was a little more than he actually was. Let's just say that, in my opinion, he thought a lot of himself—and little about me.

One of the first things he and his assistant helped me do was learn how to get into a sitting position. The goal was transferring me to a wheelchair. It was explained to me that the first step was to get me into a sitting position in the recliner located at the right side of my bed. It was an older-looking chair, dark brown and well worn. During my two months in the room, I'd seen it used often by visitors and occasional staff members with no complaints about the comfort level it provided. I had never seen it reclined, however, and this was to be where I discovered a problem with both the chair and the therapist.

The method they chose to get me into the chair was something I'd learn to utilize well over the next few months. It was a transfer board. A simple wooden board about thirty inches long and maybe eight inches wide. It had two cutouts, one on each end, which served as handles. One end was placed on the edge of my bed and the other on the seat area of the chair. The chair was at a slightly lower level than the bed, so the idea was to somehow get my butt on the thing and then use it as a sideways sliding board to get me into the chair. This sounds simple, but believe me, the first few times I tried, it was quite difficult. First of all, I didn't even have the strength to sit up on my own yet; so a couple of people were required to help get me started, one on either side of me. Once I was sitting up in the bed, I had to wiggle over to get on the board. Again, no small feat, but

I finally got it accomplished. Now I had to endeavor to press down on the board with my hands—which still had the fingers curled under, by the way—and attempt to take some weight off my butt so it could slide a couple of inches toward our target, the chair. Again, this wasn't nearly as simple as it sounds. Each movement I made had to be done with significant planning and concentration. An almost total lack of strength was something I'd never dealt with before. I'd never encountered a challenge like it. After a short time, which seemed like a long time to me, I was finally in the chair sitting straight up. I felt empowered. I had sat up in the bed before, but the bed was powered. It was adjustable, so it did all the work; but I had done this all on my own. Well, I had a little help. It hit me that this was the first time I had sat upright in a chair in almost four months. Another mountain climbed.

My elation didn't last long.

The next step was to place the chair in its reclining position. I didn't have the strength to do this, so someone else had to operate the manual switch that reclined the chair. It was when the chair was reclined that the problems started.

Remember, I said that the chair looked to be quite worn. Well, that observation turned out to be correct. Upon reclining, I immediately felt springs pop up to meet my butt and lower back. It wasn't all that uncomfortable at first, but since my back and bottom were very tender from lying flat for a long time, the discomfort quickly turned into out-and-out pain. I visualized the inner workings of the chair trying with all their might to kick me out. I could see a porcupine backed into its den, trying to fight off a bear, its quills with their razor points ready to pierce anything they encountered. The chair was the porcupine and I was the bear. And the best I can remember this scene ever playing out in the movies had the porcupine always prevailing. The bear never had a chance.

Any satisfaction I had in getting from bed to chair flew right out the window. My ass was hurting, and I expressed this to my therapist, who suddenly turned into my evil therapist. He informed me that I needed to get used to it and I was to stay in this position for forty-five minutes. I complained again, but this too fell on deaf ears as Evil Therapist turned and left the room, turning only to inform the nurses of the time I was to be returned to my bed.

I couldn't believe what was going on. I tried wiggling around as best I could and alleviated the pain for a short time, but it came back in a couple of minutes. I tried talking the nurses into helping me back to my bed—or at least to put the chair into an upright position. Even though I could tell they were somewhat sympathetic to my plight, they were clearly afraid to disobey Evil Therapist's orders. Finally, after forty-five minutes, and not a moment sooner, the nurses helped me back to my bed. I stretched out on my back and let out a sigh of utter relief. It was the kind of feeling you get when you've just completed a distance race. The pain is gone. It only gets better from here.

This scenario played out every day for a week. Oh, how I dreaded this time each day! I would watch the therapist walking in the hall and think, *Boy I hope he forgets about me today!* He never did. I grew to hate both that chair and him. Oh, how I wished I could strap him into that chair! Recline it. Laugh at him and walk off, relishing the look of sheer agony I'd see etched onto his face when I casually returned at my leisure a good while later.

The next exercise wasn't as painful, but it was no walk in the park either. It involved getting me onto a flat table mounted on a mechanism that allowed it to be tilted manually. It had straps for my ankles and a longer strap to go around my chest. Imagine Frankenstein on the operating table and you get the idea. Instead of using a transfer board, an inflatable gadget helped to move me from a gurney onto the table. The therapist rolled me over on my side and placed the inflatable thing on the table. He rolled me back onto it and switched it on. After it was inflated, it worked much like an air hockey game—with me being the puck. It was actually kind of cool. Next, I was moved onto the table and the reverse sequence of actions was executed so I was in full contact with the Frankenstein table. I was strapped down, and the table was tilted up a little and then a little more. This was quite painful, but I had already decided that I was not going to give in and seem weak to Evil Therapist.

The object of this exercise was getting my legs used to some weight bearing. When the table was at the proper angle, I was to attempt some mini-squats. The first day I couldn't, but I did a little better each successive day. Finally, on the fourth day, I had drawn a crowd for my exercise. My friend Duane was visiting that day and I had two or three nurses watching, as well as, of course, the therapists. I couldn't disappoint my audience; so once they had me in position, with great effort and a grimace on my face, I knocked out about ten three- or four-inch squats. Everybody applauded and told me just how great I'd done.

Evil Therapist then said, "I know how hard that was. You did great."

I looked him right in the eye and the words just popped out of my mouth. "Buddy, I watched my Mama and Daddy work over forty years in the cotton mill in order to raise a family. Compared to that, this is a piece of cake!"

Evil Therapist didn't give me much of a problem the rest of the short time I had left at St. Joseph's.

***

The term I began hearing more and more was rehabilitation, and this was music to my ears. Medical treatment was a phrase being tossed around a lot less. I had waited a long time to focus on getting back to normal as opposed to just surviving. As I look back on it now, it was truly a step-by-step process. I've pointed out several times that my mind, when faced with a true dilemma, seems to revert to this process; and it appeared that my body had also somehow acquired this trait along the way.

The doctors told me that my body, for the most part, had stabilized so it was possible to start, for lack of a better term, rebuilding it. And believe me, based on the loss of strength and mobility I had suffered, this was going to be a total rebuild from the ground up. But you also better believe that I was ready to get started as quickly as possible!

A case manager was assigned to me, and she explained the process from here on out. The first step would be transferring me to a rehabilitation facility, as St. Joseph's and Mission weren't set up for this. She asked if I had any facilities in mind, and I told her that I did. I was lucky enough to have a lifelong friend who was a successful physical therapist. He had recently paid me a visit and we had talked about this very subject. He told me that the most revered rehab facility in the

Southeast was in Atlanta, so that one was at the top of my list. I also asked him about anything around Charlotte and he suggested a possibility there as well. The reason I was interested in Charlotte was so I could be near my dear friend Tonya, who lived and worked there. Wherever I was to be transferred would depend upon approval from my insurance company, which in this case was Blue Cross Blue Shield of North Carolina. My caseworker told me that she'd inquire about these possibilities and get back to me the next day.

The next day she gave me the disappointing news that neither of my choices would be supported by my Blue Cross coverage. I asked if we could investigate something in the general area so it wouldn't be too difficult for my friends to visit. She said she'd compile a list and get back to me again.

The following day she came in with the options we had discussed. When she came into my room, already there were my friends Duane and Deb, who coincidently had stopped by to visit. A couple of other nurses were also in the room. She handed me the list. It contained the names of four facilities, three of which I recognized. They were all what I quantify as being nursing homes. Now, I must point something out that's essential in regard to understanding the next statement I made to her.

In 1991 a very good friend of Duane's and mine, Bruce Roland, had been involved in a near-fatal automobile accident. The accident left Bruce paralyzed from the upper part of his chest down. He could still speak and move his head and use his arms and hands, and his internal organs still operated fairly well, but that was about all. Unlike my paralysis, Bruce's was permanent. He spent a lengthy time in Carolina's Medical Center in Charlotte before being discharged and allowed to go home, where he eventually lived on his own with the assistance of home-healthcare professionals. Bruce remained on his own for several years but eventually deteriorated and ended up being transferred to a nursing facility. He was admitted to a facility very near to the area where we had all grown up. This was in the early 2000s. Duane and I visited Bruce often during his stay there, but Bruce finally passed away from natural causes in July 2010. In all the times we went to visit Bruce, I can honestly say that I witnessed very little rehabilitation taking place. Bruce was past the point of being able to respond to any rehab, but I never even saw it come into play with any of the other residents. Even though the facility appeared to be clean, I was always taken aback by the smell I encountered upon walking through the main entrance. It reeked of death and I always saw it as just place to go to die.

The next statement that jumped out of my mouth before I had a chance to come up with a more eloquent phrase was, "I ain't going to no fucking nursing home!" My case-worker told me that I might not have many more options, to which I replied, "If that's the case I'll check myself out of here and he'll (nodding toward Duane) give me a ride home!"

After getting calmed down, I explained the reason for my response. We all proceeded to have a civil conversation regarding my options, and she said she'd try to come up with a better choice.

A day or two later she informed me of a facility in Asheville only five minutes from where we sat. CarePartners would accept my insurance. I had actually been to CarePartners a few years earlier when I'd gone with a friend to visit her father, who was there recovering from a stroke. I remember being highly impressed, as it reminded me more of a hotel than any type of hospital. I don't know why we hadn't discussed this possibility before; but once we had I enthusiastically voiced my approval, and in just a couple of days I found myself saying goodbye to all the friends I'd made during my two months at St. Joseph's—a period that I'll always remember. I will always treasure my time there as the two months that saved my life.

CHAPTER SIXTEEN

JOHNNY PAYCHECK

Something I'll always remember was one of the first times I ever had to handle a severe situation that arose in the blink of an eye. I was on the spot and I had to make a decision—all the while aware that I'd never know what would have taken place had I done it differently. I just had to take the ball and run with it.

Back in 1981 and '82, I made my living in the illustrious position of bouncer and bartender at one of our area's *fine dining establishments*, the Main Street Music Hall. Main Street was centrally located between New York and Miami in the lovely town of Morganton, North Carolina, about twenty minutes from my home.

Alright, the term fine dining establishment may be a bit of a misnomer. Actually, it's an out-and-out fictitious description. Main Street was mainly a bar that featured musical acts—from all genres—and also happened to serve food. In North Carolina at the time, if you sold alcohol for on-premises consumption, you also had to serve food—and food sales had to make up at least 51 percent of your overall business.

And let's face it, that 51 percent was an out-and-out ficti-tious figure as well. Somehow, the state Alcoholic Beverage Control (ABC) Commission would not dig all that deep into your financial records back then, especially if your business was owned by one of the area's leading attorneys of the bar association, which Main Street was.

Main Street was a music hall in the truest sense of the term. It was a really nice nightclub with multi-level seating on the main floor and a multi-level balcony as well. It had originally been built and operated as a movie theater, opening in 1929; but it was closed for many years before being renovated as a disco club during the height of the disco dance era in the late '70s by my friend Bracey and another gentleman. It was named Showcase 29 and was quite successful until the demise of disco in the early '80s. That's when Bracey leased it out to a local attorney, who changed the format once more. We featured all types of live music, pretty much seven nights a week. Rock, country, rhythm and blues—you name it, we had it. We nor-mally featured local and regional acts but occasionally booked national acts as well . . . and the point of this story revolves around the night that one of these national acts was booked and what happened right in the middle of his performance.

It was a Saturday night in March of 1982 and country music superstar Johnny Paycheck was our featured artist. Most people recall Johnny Paycheck because of his enormous hit "Take This Job and Shove It." He was arguably the biggest name we'd ever had the pleasure of presenting. We had a sell-out crowd of over 500 patrons and the show started on time—but almost didn't happen at all. It was all because of what took place as Paycheck's tour bus crossed the line of Burke County, where Morganton was the county seat.

It appears Mr. Paycheck had an outstanding warrant for his arrest from the state of Utah for illicit relations with a young lady who happened not to be quite of legal age at the time of these relations. The bus was pulled over and he was served with the warrant but wasn't arrested. I never did find out how this was all arranged; at any rate, that same tour bus pulled up to the stage entrance right on time—and the 500-plus inside never knew a thing about it. What they would remember forever would happen a short time later.

On this night, I was not only working as a bouncer, but also helping out behind the bar, which I did on many overly busy nights. We had two bars. The smaller bar in front of the kitchen window was normally handled by just one person. The main bar about twenty feet across the way was large enough to accommodate three or four bartenders at the same time. I was behind the main bar when, about halfway through Paycheck's set, a former employee of the club approached me hurriedly. The expression on his face and the look in his eyes was one of both panic and dread. What he told me placed those same terrible feelings in my heart and my mind. He said, "Danny, there's a guy over there who has a gun! I just saw it!"

I asked him where exactly, and he pointed toward the small kitchen bar. Several people stood in this area, but three guys standing in a tight group somehow caught my eye. For some reason, they just looked like the type. You gain the ability to size up people quickly when you're in that business.

I saw this as an especially dangerous situation, so I didn't take the time to walk around to the exit of my bar. I went over the top and proceeded toward the three individuals. After just a few steps, an important question popped into my mind: *Dan, if you get over there and one of them does have a gun, what are you going to do about it?* The old saying, "You don't bring a knife (well, in my case it was brass knuckles) to a gun fight" immediately entered my train of thought.

The alternative that popped into my mind turned out to be crucial to how the situation turned out. We had escorted four or five people out already that night. Nothing big—just guys who had too much to drink too early and were getting a little loud and belligerent. I had taken the last fellow out myself about five minutes earlier, and we were met on the sidewalk by a couple of Morganton police officers. I talked to them and told them that the guy had had a little too much and his friend, who was also with us, was going to give him a ride home. Remembering this, I figured it would be a wise move to go out there first and see if the cops were still outside. I did—and they were, thank goodness.

I went right up to them and said, "Guys, I think we've got a guy in here with a gun."

They didn't hesitate. One officer just said, "Let's go back in, and you show us who it is."

We walked into the lobby, which was separated from the main seating level by three large archways. I was in front with the officers behind me, one off each shoulder. As soon as I got to the archway on the right, I spotted the three guys, and sure enough, the one on the left had the handle of a pistol hanging out of the right side pocket of his zip-up hooded sweatshirt. We were ten to fifteen feet away from them, but they hadn't noticed us.

I turned and told the cop to my right, "Look, there it is. It's in his pocket!"

At that very moment, the guy pulled the pistol out of his pocket, pointed it, and fired two shots. I ducked behind one of the archways and felt the two officers brush past me. In a couple of seconds, I stuck my head out and saw the cops already had the guy on the ground. I went straight to them, and as I was standing over the guy, I immediately recognized that he still had the gun in his right hand, which one of the cops had pinned to the floor, his foot on the guy's wrist. The other cop had his gun drawn, pointing right between the man's eyes while at the same time loudly ordering him, "Drop the gun!! Drop the gun!!"

The fellow stated, "Don't kill me. I did what I wanted to do." He immediately dropped the gun.

All hell proceeded to break loose. People were running all over the place, screaming and yelling. I ran behind the bar and grabbed the baseball bat that I regularly carried with me when walking to and from my vehicle each night. I didn't know the reason for what had just transpired, and I wanted to be safe. I noticed a group of people gathered near the center aisle on the second level in front of the stage. I rushed over and saw a man lying face down with a woman standing over him screaming and crying hysterically. I started clearing the area, and immediately police officers swarmed the place. They really had gotten there in record time. Shortly, we had the building cleared except for those who had been identified as potential witnesses. After the coroner arrived, when they rolled the victim over, I got to see the effect that a .357 round has on the human body. Both shots had struck him. One had entered his lower back and exited his left leg, and the other had struck him squarely in the middle of his back, exiting the center of his chest. That exit wound was probably the size of a grapefruit. The sight was unnerving. Like something out of a horror movie—except this time, I was in the movie.

The entire episode turned out to be a jealous exhusband scenario that played out all too often back then. I won't go into the details, but the exhusband was finally tried and found guilty (I testified in the trial) and received a sentence of seven to ten years for premeditated murder. Unfortunately, back then in this part of the country, light sentences for a crime so severe also played out all too often.

I spent the rest of the night down at the police station answering questions and writing statements. I felt terrible about the fact that a man had just died inside the place where it was my job to keep people safe. However, just before I left, the officer who had been assigned to stay with me told me something that gave me at least a small amount of solace regarding my actions on that fateful night. He looked me right in the eye and said, "Dan, if you hadn't reacted the way you did tonight, things could have been much worse."

As I look back on it, I realize that this was the first time in my life when I was faced with a life-or-death situation. Little did I know that many more were to come as time wore on. Severe situations will occur in all our lives. It seems to me that I was even lucky to encounter these happenings a bit more often than others in order to tell my story. Whatever the case, they did come my way, and I'm living proof that they can be dealt with if you have the correct mindset. It will work. Perseverance is the key. Don't ever think that there's nothing you can do about a bad situation. Nothing is inevitable. You can always deal with any situation. Just keep on keeping on. Keep the faith, Brother. Retain that faith in yourself. You'll come out on top; and even if things go south, always remember that you did the best you could.

CHAPTER SEVENTEEN

CAREPARTNERS

On January 3, 2016, I was wheeled out of my room at St. Joseph's for the last time. Still in my bed, I was taken around to say goodbye to all the staff on duty that morning. I can honestly say that the term *mixed emotions* isn't sufficient to describe the feelings I experienced. I was extremely excited to check into a rehabilitative environment and leave behind the more serious medical issues. At the same time, it was sad to leave the new friends I'd made. The friendships I had made up to the point before I fell ill had all come about in the same manner: mutual interests, physical attractions, classmates, teammates, co-workers. The friendships I'd forged at St. Joseph's Hospital came into being under the direst of circumstances. When I was admitted two months earlier, I had narrowly escaped death after a six-week stint on the critical list in the Intensive Care Unit at Mission Hospital. I was improved but still depending on machines and the actions of my caregivers for my continued existence. These people had kept me alive and provided the treatment to get me to this point by this third day of a new year.

I doubt that I'll ever encounter this same set of circumstances again—at least I hope I don't—but the relationships I developed over those last two months of what had turned out to be the most challenging year of my life were, let's just say, very special. I look back and wonder if doctors and nurses feel the same way about the relationships that evolve with their patients. Surely not. The sheer number of interactions would seem to water down any chance of this possibility. But I must also believe that, occasionally, a special case might come along to cause their minds to store memories of a few particular patients in the rarely used, very secure area of their brains. Just maybe . . .

After all the goodluck wishes and more than a few tears, I was loaded into an EMS vehicle and transported about three minutes down Biltmore Avenue, then two more minutes up Sweeten Creek Road to CarePartners Rehabilitation Hospital, an eight-bed facility that had opened in 1938 as Thoms Rehabilitation Hospital. Originally, it was a facility geared toward caring for children with assorted disabilities. A multitude of pictures from this period still adorn the walls of the long hallway that connects the housing units to the auditorium and the therapy swimming pool—a hallway that I'd travel daily for the next two months.

Operating under the CarePartners | Mission Health moniker, it's now an intense rehabilitation atmosphere for adults suffering from a myriad of disabilities. When I was wheeled inside to my new surroundings, room 153, I wasn't 404 any longer. I was 153. Room 153 was actually a double room, but I never had a roommate there. It was large with an adjacent bathroom that featured, in addition to a fully handicap-equipped toilet and sink area, a shower head mounted on the opposite wall with a tile floor and drain. It reminded me of locker room showers, only more private.

On that first day, I was unable to use any of the features in that bathroom; but that would change in the following weeks. Another unusual but very practical feature was a small high definition TV mounted on a movable arm attached to the head of the bed. I could just swing the TV nearby whenever I wanted, or swing it back out of the way. As had been the case at St. Joseph's, Danny's TV was rarely turned off. It was again my bedtime companion—there for me when I awoke during the night, providing me with welcome variety to the sometimes depressing feelings that come to you only during these times when you awaken and the reality of your situation is right in front of your eyes. You can close your eyes, but it's still there in your mind. This happened often, but I could always depend on my friend, the TV, to be there for me. It never let me down.

All the staff I met on that first day seemed friendly and positive. I was impressed—and eager to get started. There was an unmistakably professional vibe to this place, and I just got a feeling that this was a place where good things happened. It was the place I needed to be, and I was ready to show that I was worthy of being there.

The feeling from that initial impression of CarePartners was one of opportunity—an opportunity for a new beginning. I'd been down a very long, rough road over the previous four months, but I'd worked hard to find the end of that road, as had all the doctors and nurses and other staff who had traveled that road with me.

I liken it to camping with only a tent for shelter when an intense thunderstorm rolls in just after nightfall. The storm keeps raging and just when you think it must let up, it only grows more commanding. You find yourself completely powerless to do anything other than hunker down and hope for the best. The storm keeps getting louder and stronger, and eventually you pass out from exhaustion. After a time, you wake to notice it's still dark, but finally the storm seems to be showing signs of weakening. Gradually the wind slows and the rain lightens; and after what seems like forever, you notice the faint glow of what must be the sun rising. It slowly grows brighter and brighter, and the woods fall silent. You eventually work up the courage to unzip the door of the tent to look at what's left of the outside world. You cast your eyes outside, expecting terrible destruction; but even though some damage is evident, you see golden rays of sunshine reflecting off the bright green leaves. The raindrops on those leaves act as prisms, amplifying the sun's rays. It's a glorious sight . . . and you realize there may be hope after all.

The analogy harkens back to an event that occurred many years ago, but one that will forever be ingrained in my mind.

After I quit the tryouts for that little league baseball team at age ten, it was one of the greatest regrets of my life. I was disgusted and demoralized. I spent a few weeks feeling sorry for myself; and then I decided I'd get to work to make myself into a better ball player so when tryout time came the next year, I'd make my Daddy proud and get a little personal satisfaction as well.

I spent countless hours practicing. Everything from throwing a tennis ball off a concrete wall and having it bounce back to me so I could improve my arm and my fielding at the same time, to hitting acorns Daddy would throw to me in the backyard during the fall and fielding ground balls he'd hit to me. Back in those days, kids actually stayed after school and played pickup games down on the ballfield where I had disgraced myself just a few months prior. It was the only baseball field where I'd ever played. Just a sandlot, more or less, but a baseball field just the same.

I worked hard. Very hard. But I always had the feeling that when springtime came and tryouts were scheduled, I would again not live up to my own expectations. I tried to push this thought away; and even though it may have diminished, it still persisted. I never gave up though. Even in the dead of winter when it was much too cold to practice much of the game, you could usually find me outside after school with a bat, at least practicing my swing. I knew I might fail again, but this time it wouldn't be because I didn't try.

Around the end of May, the time finally came, and all us kids gathered to see who'd make the team. Lo and behold—not only did I make it, I earned a starting position at first base. Things were looking up.

Finally, the day came for our first game, a home game. On this biggest of days, my mom had washed my uniform and laid it all out on my bed. I still remember putting on that old felt uniform for the first time. First, I put on a pair of white tube socks, then pulled up the blue-and-white striped stirrup socks over them. Next came the white pants that reached just below the knee, a white T-shirt with three-quarter-length blue sleeves, and finally my jersey, which featured piping around the neck and down the button line with NEBO across the front chest and number 15 boldly emblazoned on the back. This ritual would be repeated countless times over the next several years. Always in the same order. The only things that would change were the lettering on the front and—with a couple of teams along the way—the number on the back.

I don't remember if my dad gave me a ride to that first game or if I walked, but I do remember vividly what I would encounter when I got to the field.

Our Nebo field had been transformed into the Nebo Ball park. The all-dirt infield had been smoothed out and raked in a circular fashion. There wasn't a bad spot on it. It was immaculate. The baselines and batter's boxes were laid out with wide, bright, white chalk. The bases were strapped down at exactly sixty-foot lengths, with those baselines running precisely along the inside edges. The pitcher's rubber looked like the bright white sanitary center of the entire infield— and all that was to come would emanate from it. The outfield grass was bright green and mowed close to the ground. And seemed to go on forever, as our field didn't have an outfield fence. But, in right field it did have a barrier of sorts. It had the bank that I'd walked up just a year before when I shame- fully left this same field. If I'd ever walk up that bank this year, it would be at the conclusion of a game—and I would be wearing a uniform.

Our coach finally yelled for all of us to gather at our bench, which was on the first-base side. He read off the opening-day lineup and batting order. I was hitting fourth. The clean-up spot. He told us it was time to get out there for a little round of infield practice before the game. I grabbed my first-baseman's mitt and ran toward my position—and abruptly stopped right at the first-base line. I didn't want to step onto that perfectly manicured playing field. I didn't want to disturb its perfec- tion. Its beauty. Its holiness.

I knew I'd be stepping into something unknown. I pondered that fact for what seemed like hours, but I'm sure it was only seconds. Many things ran through my mind, much of which was my recollection of quitting the previous year and how hard I had worked to earn the right to step across that line. A feeling of confidence eventually came over me. I took that first step into the unknown; I've never regretted that step for one second, and I've never looked back.

My first day at CarePartners wasn't unlike that first day on the field. They gave me a standard orientation to my new surroundings. However, three things stand out as being especially satisfying. One, I was getting a motorized wheelchair. This opened important possibilities. Something we all take for granted, until it's no longer available to us, is the freedom to move about. I spent my entire two months at St. Joseph's confined to my room. Occasionally someone would wheel me to other areas for tests, but during the last few days they would help me into a wheelchair and push me into the hall near the nurse's station. Then I'd pick out a spot just a few floor tiles away and do my best to roll myself there. My fingers were still curled up, and I wasn't yet able to grip the circular handrail on the outside of each wheel, so what little strength I had in my arms was no aid in propelling myself either forward or backward. When I was able to roll myself just five or six feet, I gained a huge feeling of satisfaction; and I'm sure the nurses tired of hearing about my accomplishments.

I also consider how much I had taken for granted being able to go outside anytime I wanted. I've always been an outdoors kind of person, and to have that taken away was demoralizing. The two narrow windows in my room were the only link I'd had with the outdoors for eight weeks. Those two windows were just off to my right side, and I can't tell you how many hours I spent gazing out, wishing I could be out there walking around where my eyes could see.

It occurred to me that this must be what prisoners experience in segregation housing. But wait, even they get to go outside a few times a week for short recreation sessions, even if they're in full restraints. My God, I had it worse than a convict. I didn't even get outside rec . . . except for the day I was able to talk one of the assistant physical therapists into taking me outside. One afternoon, this young girl with long, frizzy brown hair helped me into my chair and took me to the elevator. We went down to the lobby and she proceeded to push me through the automatic doors into the outside world! That first breath of fresh air after four months felt absolutely purifying in my lungs. I took another deep breath, then another, another, another. I couldn't get enough. It was especially cold that day in December and the cold, crisp mountain air felt better than any breaths I had ever taken in my life. Because of the cold temperatures, my dear enabler would let me stay outside for only a few minutes; but believe me, they were a few minutes that I'll always treasure.

After I demonstrated that I could adequately operate my motorized wheelchair, which I caught on to quickly, I was able to navigate to daily therapy sessions on my own. Once they helped me get my butt into it in the morning, I didn't get back into the bed most days until it was time to go to sleep. I had my run of the joint. Hell, I was back on the road again, so to speak. That feeling returned many months later when I finally started driving a car again. Freedom to move about is not something to be taken lightly, my friends.

The second satisfying thing they told me the first day in rehab was that I'd no longer have to wear a hospital gown. I could wear my own clothes. The very next day my friend Duane was nice enough to bring me a selection of T-shirts, sweatshirts, gym shorts, and tennis shoes from my extensive collection at home.

I looked at this as a major step toward regaining my independence. Getting a little further toward recapturing the ol' Danny, who I'd lost, at least partly, over the previous several months.

When I got off work around 5:00 each day, I'd head straight to the Y for my daily workout. I would go directly to the locker room and change into a T-shirt. It always gave me a great sense of relief to get out of my work attire, which was usually business casual—sometimes even with a shirt and tie. Changing was like a breath of fresh air. Quite liberating. I could leave the events of the day behind and just concentrate on getting a good workout and, of course, subsequently improving my health. When I was allowed to wear my clothes again, I realized that putting them on each morning would help me forget about the events of the previous four months and focus on physically getting back to some semblance of who I used to be. This was extremely comforting.

The third and last satisfying thing came when it was explained to me that, after an initial evaluation, I'd be placed on a structured schedule. It would change somewhat from day to day but would, for the most part, take up my entire day. The key word here is *structured*. As I've mentioned, I have always found that I'm one of those people who benefit from structure. My confidence level rises significantly when I have a well-thought-out, structured schedule to adhere to. And as my confidence level goes up, so does my productive output. Inhibitions go right out the window and positivity comes right in through the front door. The biggest difference, however, would be that this structured schedule wasn't authored by me. Others would put it together. This concerned me a bit at first, but after just a few days I gained a tremendous amount of respect for those in charge of my care and recovery. They knew what the hell they were doing. I could read that fact like a book. I put my complete confidence in these people; and this, in turn, put me in a tunnel-vision mode of getting better as quickly as possible. I was told several times before I arrived at CarePartners that they'd work me hard every day, so I needed to be ready for it. Hey, that's exactly what I wanted, and it was exactly what I got. I realized that I needed to cram in as much of this level of rehabilitation as possible in the shortest amount of time as possible because I knew Blue Cross wasn't going to pick up the tab any longer than they had to. I was ready to get at it!

After my initial evaluation, my first weekday at CarePartners served as a blueprint of sorts for what I was to expect each day. Promptly at 7:20 AM, at least one nurse would come in and wake me if I wasn't already up, always with a smile and a positive attitude. I've never been a morning person, but I must say, during my two months' stay I started to become one; and I know I owed it all to just two factors. Number one was that pleasant awakening each morning, and number two was my own expectation of what the day would bring and how much I could accomplish.

The first order of business was to check out the schedule for the day, which was delivered sometime between 4:00 a.m.

(when I was also awakened for my scheduled medication) and the 7:20 get-up-and-get-going ritual. I never saw the person who left this schedule, but a fresh one appeared each morning, usually taped to the back of my electric wheelchair. It was kind of like Santa Claus coming on Christmas morning when I was a kid. I never got to see him in the flesh, but there were always presents under the tree—so somebody had to have left them. Santa or my parents? I had suspicions, but no actual proof. Same thing here. Could have been a nurse, but could have been the daily schedule fairy as well. Again, suspicions, but no actual proof.

The next activity was eating breakfast, which I had selected from a menu on the previous day. I ate almost the same thing for breakfast every day. Just as I had before this ordeal unfolded and I was still a (somewhat) normal person, I had some go-to breakfast foods. They were things I liked, and I stuck with them for extended periods until I finally grew tired of the same thing every day. My selections from the CarePartners menu were usually centered around Cinnamon Toast Crunch™ cereal with a banana cut up in it, swimming in a milk bath that was as big as a small carton of milk could create. My routine also included not one but two fruit cups, cut-up cantaloupe and honeydew, along with grapes and sometimes pineapple; a small container of apple juice, one of orange juice, and another carton of milk. Occasionally, on the weekend, I'd change up and go with bacon or link sausage with scrambled eggs and toast; but the cereal start to the day remained my favorite for Monday through Friday, or the "work week" which, for all intents and purposes, these days turned out to be for me.

As I look back on it now, I realize that my breakfast selections mirrored what I ate when growing up. On weekdays Mama always fixed something quick and nourishing, but on the weekend, she amplified things a little on Saturday with pancakes—and blew the roof off on Sunday with eggs, grits, biscuits and gravy, sausage, bacon, and many times, country ham with red-eye gravy. I'll never forget waking up and smelling these things cooking. I ascertained the day of the week by the smells coming from the kitchen. I guess I never outgrew it.

The number one thing that was special about my breakfast was that it had to be fed to me by a nurse. I was still unable to feed myself. I learned on this first day that it was one of the prime issues to be addressed during my daily occupational therapy sessions. As I've mentioned previously, when you go through an event as drastic as this, you must totally depend on those around you for every iota of your existence, and therefore, you lose all pride along the way. If you'd have asked me just six months before how I imagine it would feel to have to be fed breakfast by a twenty-one-year-old girl with long blond hair, I'd have said it would be demeaning. Not anymore, Brother! The nurse normally on duty at this time was indeed a beautiful young blond with a very pleasing personality, and I didn't have any problem whatsoever with her feeding me every spoonful of my morning meal. I looked forward to seeing her every morning. But I did vow to myself that, before I left this place—even though I'd still be happy for her to wake me each morning—she wouldn't have to feed me any longer. I'd show her I could perform this most elemental duty on my own.

Another area that was demeaning early on, but about which I had absolutely no concern whatsoever by this point, was having to be dressed by another person—and 90 percent of the time, someone of the opposite sex. Because I was no longer required to wear a hospital gown, the second exercise of the day was to get Dan into a pair of shorts and a T-shirt. I was still unable to do this myself and was even farther away from the next step, which was putting on a pair of socks and tennis shoes. I'd proudly get past the shorts-and-shirt threshold before I was discharged, but the socks-and-shoes barrier was something I wouldn't cross until several months down the road.

After dressing, I needed to brush my teeth and comb my hair. That's right, all you fans out there in radio land, I couldn't pull off these tasks either. Sounds incredible, but I refer again to my analogy of being like a little baby. I had to learn how to do everything all over again. My mind knew how to perform these tasks just as it always had. The old body just wasn't giving me a lot of cooperation and support.

After these daily morning duties were conquered, the final task in the friendly confines of room 153 was the old transfer from bed to wheelchair. It was awfully difficult at first, but I improved fairly quickly and was able to do it on my own within a few weeks. When I was finally in the chair, I was off on my own for my first appointment of the day. Swimming pool therapy!

My room was near one end of the CarePartners facility, and the therapy pool was situated at the opposite end. So, my little ride over there every morning gave me a chance to say good morning to a lot of people as I passed the nurses' stations and arrived at the occupational therapy section. Then it was a lengthy ride down a quiet, solitary hallway lined with photographs depicting the hospital's beginning days when it was still a children's rehab facility run largely by nuns. These photos were very interesting to me, and I tried to get an early start each morning so I'd have a little time to take in all these images from days gone by and still be on time for my appointment at the pool. Many of the pictures were quite touching. I tried to put myself into the places of the children featured in each shot. Even though I was handicapped just as the kids in the photos were, I never was able to fully identify with them, since I was an adult who'd already been through many trials and tribulations in my life that they had not.

The way I saw it, I was much more prepared for the tough road ahead; and I just couldn't imagine being in their individual situations. My God, it must have been an incredible challenge for them, not having before been tested. In most cases, being handicapped was all they'd ever known. I tried every day to somehow put myself into their shoes but never was fully able to do so.

At the end of the photo area, the hallway took a left turn and went up a short incline, and finally I found myself at the entrance to the pool area. The pool therapy section was run by a crew of three. Reta, in her mid-thirties, was the certified therapist and henceforth, the manager. She had two assistants who were both doing their physical therapy internships: Lee from the Northeast and Megan from central North Carolina— both in their twenties.

All three were attractive, healthy individuals with tremendous personalities and very positive attitudes. We hit it off on our first meeting and I genuinely feel, as time went on, that we grew eager to see each other at the beginning of each day. At least, it sure felt that way to me.

The first order of business was to get me changed into appropriate swimming pool attire, which, in my case, amounted to different shorts and tennis shoes. The reason for wearing the shoes rather than going barefoot was that the soles of my feet had become very tender from nonuse and were easily cut by anything resembling an abrasive surface, which did (slightly) exist on the bottom of the old concrete and tile pool bottom.

I still needed a lot of help transferring from my chair over to the flat changing table against the left wall of the dressing room. It took everything Lee and Megan had to get me over there in the first place, and then getting me rolled back and forth and changed. It was no small feat but it, as well as everything else, got easier and more manageable as the days passed.

Once I was changed, the next endeavor was to transfer me into a wheelchair made of PVC pipe with a seat made of web mesh. Then they'd roll me out of the dressing room and through a door that opened to the pool where Reta was waiting. The pool itself was probably half the size of an Olympic pool with a ramp at the shallow end that zig-zagged back and forth toward deeper water. The maximum depth was about five feet.

I vividly remember the first time Reta rolled me onto that ramp and into the water. The sensation of that warm water hitting my feet and then covering my ankles, then my calves, my knees, then the bottom of my thighs and butt until I was underwater from the waist down and facing the deep end. I had not been in a bathtub or shower since September. It was January. It felt absolutely heavenly. I could have sat right there for the rest of the day and been perfectly happy. Maybe with the daily paper to read and possibly some hot dogs to munch on and Cokes to drink . . . I would have been content. But lo and behold, the best was yet to come.

Reta stepped around to the front of the chair, took my hands . . . and told me to stand up. Now you've got to remember that I hadn't stood on my own two feet since September; so her direction to stand was met in my mind by great anticipation—but a fair amount of trepidation as well. I wanted so badly to stand up, but could I actually do it? I didn't know. I really, really wanted to, but I just didn't know. *Well, hell, here goes.*

I did it. I was standing.

I was actually standing. I felt ten feet tall. I have never felt liberation as strongly as I did that morning in January 2016; and I doubt that I ever will again.

The water was holding me up, and as Reta led me farther into the deeper water where Lee and Megan waited, it supported me that much more. What an incredible sensation! The physical sense of being enveloped in this perfectly clear and radiantly warm water that had just a hint of a chlorine scent— combined with the massive head rush of being able to stand again—was probably the best beginning to a day I'd ever had. Hard to top that, indeed.

This was the ritual we would perform each day. Get me changed, get me into the pool—and then the real therapy would start. They'd have me do various exercises centered around balance and coordination, which were quite challenging at first but got easier each day, just as they were supposed to. In the beginning I'd have to hold someone's hand as a

AIN'T DEAD YET • 135

centering point even to take a step, but eventually I could just hold onto the side of the pool . . . and finally I could walk and carry out the exercises without holding on to anything. As I look back on it now, I really believe the pool therapy over those two months did more to build my confidence than anything else I did at CarePartners.

Another benefit of the hour I spent with Reta, Lee, and Megan every day was the conversation. All three were easy to talk to, and I believe they really looked forward to what I had to say. I've never been afraid to share my thoughts on pretty much any subject, and I found that, after going through what I had been through, any inhibitions that remained had utterly disappeared. It really seemed that they got a lot of enjoyment out of conversing with someone who wasn't afraid to express his opinion and share his history, as opposed to the normal banter they'd have with more conservative patients during the course of a day.

Those conversations, along with the looks they'd give each other when I pulled off some new, difficult exercise, are two things I'll never forget about those sessions.

Many times, the next thing on my daily schedule after pool therapy was a visit to one of the in-house psychiatrists. It initially bothered me that I was scheduled for this type of appointment. I mean, I had been through a tremendous amount physically over several months, but I still considered myself mentally competent. I'd never received any type of psychiatric treatment in my life, nor had I ever considered myself a candidate for such. However, I wasn't about to refuse to attend. Things were going too well to take a chance on upsetting the momentum. Besides, I thought it might be interesting, and I may even learn something. So, I maneuvered my big electric wheelchair into the mental health area right on schedule.

The doctor assigned to my case seemed to be a nice enough fellow. He was probably in his fifties with close-cut hair and eyeglasses. Don't all psychiatrists wear glasses? That's the way they're always portrayed on TV and in the movies. This guy looked as if he could have stepped into any of those roles I'd seen on the screen. After we got the normal initial pleasantries out of the way, I decided to cut right to the chase and proceeded to ask him, "Just why am I here?"

His answer made a lot of sense, and I felt downright stupid for not having realized this fact on my own. A fellow who's been through traumatic illness or a physical event to a degree that would require the rehabilitation provided by this facility likely would suffer severe mental injuries when he realized the condition he was in and considered the prognosis of his case, which may be bleak at best.

I've often said that the most unaddressed illnesses in the world today are mental illnesses. It is fascinating to me that, in this day and age, mental issues are still in many instances the red-headed stepchild of society. Too many people want to look the other way and just pretend that the condition doesn't exist. One thing I've had the chance to experience firsthand due to my varied life experiences is meeting people from all walks of life. I can assure you that mental illness is very much a horrible reality. It can destroy one's existence from the inside out. I've seen it too many times. And now that I've had a chance to see human existence from a different perspective, I realize why it most certainly could manifest itself in the rehab environment, especially in the form of severe depression. I've been asked many times how I was able to keep my spirits up, and I wish I could answer that question. Maybe it's something in my makeup, something from how I was raised, things I'd experienced. I really don't know.

My mental health professional and I hit it off well. During our first few meetings he went through the normal protocol questioning for evaluation purposes; but as we progressed, I found that we were spending most of our hour just talking about everyday things. Current events, common interests, things of that nature.

One day I showed up for my appointment a few minutes early and my doctor wasn't there yet, so I decided to have a little fun. I maneuvered myself into his rather tight, cramped office, turned myself around, and backed into a position (somewhat) behind his desk. He hurriedly walked in just a few minutes later, and before he had a chance to survey the situation or utter a single word, I said, "Hi, Doc. Good to see you. How are things going today? Have a seat."

To my surprise, he sat down in one of the two cushioned chairs in front of his desk and said, "Sorry I'm late, but I've been so rushed today. I really don't know which end's up." To which, I responded:

"Well, just take a deep breath and tell me about it."

He actually started to take that breath when he finally reaized what was playing out. He laughed. "Well, a little role reversal exercise, huh?"

We both had a big chuckle, switched places, and finished our visit. For some reason, that turned out to be the last mental health appointment to show up on my daily schedule. Guess I was looked upon as being cured.

My first activity after lunch break each day was occupational therapy. Two therapists were assigned to my case,

Dawn and Michelle. Both were young ladies, probably in their thirties, with outstanding personalities. Initially, Michelle was the therapist I saw on most days, but eventually the two would alternate as to who would see me on any particular day. I didn't care which one I had. I liked both. I really looked forward to our five-day-per-week sessions, which convened at 1:00 PM each afternoon.

The first thing Michelle took on was the task of straightening out my fingers so I could use my hands more effectively. She made braces that fit on the underside of each forearm and extended over my palms and onto the tips of my fingers. The braces were fashioned from a plastic material that was placed into a bath of very hot water, making it somewhat pliable. She shaped it to fit each forearm and hand—a process that was painstaking, requiring multiple fittings and filling almost three complete, one-hour sessions. When they were finally finished, I took them back to my room, and when bedtime rolled around, the night nurse would set them in place by wrapping an elastic ace bandage from each elbow to the tips of my fingers. With the bandage entirely in place, my fingers were completely straightened out. The braces stayed in place until morning, when they were removed by the first-shift nurses. At first I couldn't see much improvement, but as time wore on, I could tell my fingers and hands were able to accomplish a little bit more each day. I know I use this phrase a lot, but you really don't know what you've got till it's gone; and the use of your hands is one of the things—if not the thing—I realized I missed the most. The use of your hands mirrors your independence within your very existence. Your hands are essential to almost everything you undertake in a normal day. Just think about it. Nearly every physical task you carry out, no matter how simple or how difficult, requires the use of your hands. They're like two friends that I now realize I had always taken for granted. It was so comforting to see these friends I had missed so much finally coming back around.

With my hands beginning to work again, the objective at the top of my list was one of the most primary in nature. I needed to learn how to feed myself again. They utilized a small, simple apparatus that had a slot forged into it that accommodated the handle of a spoon or fork. It was attached to my wrist with a simple Velcro strap. I had to learn how to maneuver it from plate to mouth without spilling what I'd managed to get into the spoon. Sounds simple enough. It wasn't. Like everything else, I had to learn from the ground up again.

I had to perform an exercise during which I used the spoon in the apparatus to pick up plastic marbles from a bowl and transfer them to a cup. Again, sounds simple. Again, it wasn't. It was so frustrating trying to get those dang little marbles from point A to point B without spilling any; but I stuck to it, and after a few days I just about had it mastered.

My crowning achievement came about four weeks in, when my dinner was delivered to my room one evening. Usually, within five minutes a nurse would come in and feed me. On this day, however, she was running a little late. I had selected stew beef with mashed potatoes and gravy and mixed vegetables. One of my favorites. All the food at CarePartners was very good, but this was one I would order every single time it was available. I took the lid off the dish. (Yes, I could do it!) Inhaled the aroma. Looked at the thing that held the spoon I'd been practicing with . . . and decided to take a shot. I was able to get the spoon thing around my wrist fairly easily and it was off to the races. It wasn't pretty, but the final outcome was deemed a success by the nurse who finally came in, apologized for being late, then took the lid off my dish only to find almost all of the food to be gone.

She asked who had come in to feed me.

I proudly replied, "I'll have you to know that I was able to help myself to today's evening meal, thank you."

She let out a high pitched, "Woooo Hoooo!" and gave me a big hug, telling me how proud she was of me.

Man, that was satisfying. From that day on, I ate every meal on my own as best I could, and I relished every bite.

This victory transferred over into other areas as Michelle and Dawn addressed them. They taught me how to brush my teeth on my own, comb my hair, dress myself, and all the rest. All those little elementary things we take for granted that had been taken away from me by Guillain-Barré were given back to me in that hospital over that two-month period. I will forever be grateful.

A lot of exceptional things ensued around the same time I took those first bites on my own. One day I was in my room between appointments, and one of the nurses came in pushing a wheelchair that looked much like the one I used during pool therapy. I asked her why she had brought my pool chair all the way over to 153.

She replied, "Don't tell anyone you've got this, okay?" She pushed it into the bathroom, closed the door, and left.

I was certainly more than a little perplexed, but since she had told me not to say anything, I thought I'd just play along. I mean, what could a plastic-frame, mesh-seat wheelchair do to hurt me anyway?

AIN'T DEAD YET • 141

That evening around 7:00, two of the second-shift nurses came in and said, "We've got a surprise for you!"

Of course, my eyes and ears perked up as one of them proceeded to open the bathroom door and bring out the mysterious new wheelchair.

She said, "We all know how much you've been wanting to take a real shower again, and tonight we're going to make that wish come true."

I'll have to admit that I had hungered for a real shower and had mentioned it several times. Since this adventure began, I had received only sponge baths. Being able to get into the pool every morning had helped with this desire greatly, but it still didn't bring total satisfaction. Remember, the bathroom in room 153 had large shower head mounted on the wall and a drain in the floor; but I was still unable to use it—or anything else in the bathroom for that matter—due to the unfortunate fact that I still was unable to walk into it.

Finally it all made sense. They were going to help me into that chair, roll me into the shower, and make me a happy guy—and that's just what they proceeded to do. In no time they had me undressed and in the chair. One of them had already turned on the showerhead, and the sound of the water hitting the tile floor was unmistakable. The sight of steam rising off the hot water as they pushed me in was akin to floating into a dream; and believe me, once the first streams of that hot, steamy water cascaded down onto my skin, I had to ask myself if I was having one of those vivid dreams again. The feeling of that water hitting the top of my head and running down my back provided a feeling that can only be defined as luxurious. At that moment, I could just as well have been in a five-star hotel in the middle of New York City rather than in a rehab hospital in Asheville, North Carolina. I felt pampered.

Since I still wasn't able to hold a slippery bar of soap, they did me the honor of bathing me. They even followed my old routine of showering, starting at the top and finishing at the bottom. They even threw in a shampoo. Outstanding. Once we were finished, they wheeled me back beside my bed and even had a blow dryer and brush ready to take care of my hair, which, by this time, was starting to get a little long. Once I was completely dried off and in a pair of shorts, they helped me get back into the bed. I don't think I have ever felt as cleansed as I did that night in February 2016. What had I done to deserve it? I felt like royalty. I thanked them over and over, and they just replied that they were proud of me for working hard and keeping a positive attitude.

The showering ritual continued to play out every other night, right up until the day I was discharged. And you know, I never did tell anyone else I had a special wheelchair in my room. Until now, that is.

Another exceptional thing happened just a few days later, when I received a visit from someone whom I certainly didn't expect but welcomed with open arms. I looked up one Sunday evening, and—lo and behold—who walked in the door but my first girlfriend, Nancy. I hadn't seen her in years. We had remained friendly but didn't stay in close contact. Nancy, who's always been a great singer, gets booked into churches, rest homes, and other venues for inspirational programs as part of her profession; and that's why she was in the area on this particular evening. She said she'd first found out about my condition from Facebook posts and had made a few calls to check on me further, and then she apologized for not having made it over to see me sooner.

She stayed with me for a little over two hours, and we never stopped talking the entire time. We had a lot of catching up to do. We covered every topic that came to mind that night except one, a topic that pops into my head anytime I see her or talk to her. It concerns something that happened almost forty years ago.

I'd been at a high school football game, and Nancy came up to me and asked if I could give her a ride home, as we lived near each other. This was before we started dating. I told her I'd be happy to. Once the game was over, we got into my 1972 Plymouth Duster and went down the road. When we got to her house, I pulled into the driveway and stopped opposite their screened-in porch, which had the light on for her, as it looked as though her parents had already gone to bed.

We talked for a while and finally she said, "Well, I guess I better go in."

I replied something to the effect of, "Yeah, I better be getting home myself."

Right at that moment, she reached over and put her hand around my neck, pulled me over to her and planted on me the first kiss that I had ever received from any girl. And not just a kiss, but a French kiss—man, did she know what she was doing! And just as quick, she let me go, got out of the car, walked up the steps, and went through the door of that screened-in porch and into her house, turning to wave goodbye just before entering.

I was stunned.

If I could have received a million dollars for saying a word—any word—right then, my income wouldn't have increased one penny. I don't remember cranking the car, driving home, or walking into the door of my house that night; but now, forty years later, I'm sure I'll forevermore remember my first kiss.

In my mind, the main bridge to be crossed during my rehab stay wasn't learning how to feed myself again, brush my teeth and hair, dress myself, or any of the other things I recovered the ability to perform while I was a patient there. No, the biggest bridge by far was regaining the ability to walk, to stand on my own two feet, to be mobile once more.

I confronted this mission during physical therapy sessions that occurred five, and occasionally six, days per week at 3:00 PM. I had three PTs assigned to my case. Daniel, Leslie, and Fred. Daniel and Leslie were both already certified physical therapists, and Fred was doing his internship. An interesting fact is that Fred's first day at CarePartners was the day I arrived, and his last day was the day I was discharged. He's now a certified physical therapist and works in his home state of Maryland.

All three were easy to get along with and seemed very knowledgeable concerning their craft. Something I noticed then that was reinforced during a return visit two years later was how all the employees in the physical therapy section got along extremely well. During that visit in March of 2018, I noticed absolutely no turnover in the staff in this section. I've always believed that a stable workforce is a good indication of a productive workforce.

Another thing I noticed was that all three were easy to talk to, as were all the people I encountered during my stay. I liken our daily conversations to those I had earlier during pool therapy. Make no mistake about it, business came first, but we found time to discuss whatever else was on our minds. Again, I fully believe they enjoyed working with someone with a little different attitude and outlook than the run-of-the-mill patients they encountered daily. Maybe that's massaging my own ego a bit, but if so, so be it. Sometimes giving your ego a little boost isn't a bad idea.

I made it clear from the start that my ultimate goal—if I got to stay with them long enough—was to walk out the front door all by myself on discharge day; and they made it clear that they'd do everything in their power to help me achieve this. And they did. They worked me hard, but not overly so. As a matter of fact, on most days I'd try to talk them into spending just a few more minutes with me, since my appointment was their last of the day; and often times, they did just that.

On February 6, 2016, just over four weeks into my stay, the staff had me ready to attempt my first steps. A device called a walking frame would be involved to provide support, but I'd be providing the power on my own. I look back on the video recorded that day, and one of the first things that impressed me was the number of people who showed up to witness my first attempt. I must have invited everybody in the hospital because there were about twenty people watching, including my friends Duane and Deb, who had driven up from home to give me support. I was truly impressed.

Initially, Fred and Leslie helped me up on my feet, positioning themselves on rolling stools on either side. They gave me verbal instruction and encouragement through my walk, which took all of one minute and six seconds. I took a total of sixteen small steps and covered twelve to fifteen feet, but to me, I had just finished a marathon. I was elated! I was on my way!

My progress continued with the walking frame as support, but I wanted so much to get away from it. I mean, you just can't carry around a fifty-pound monstrosity like that everywhere you go. Not cool at all.

Fred liked to refer to me as Jackson Daniel, my wrestling moniker—and that was alright with me. It kept the mood light.

At the conclusion of one day toward the end of February, Fred said, "Jackson Daniel, tomorrow we're going to take it up a notch and try a few steps on a walker."

Well, that next day we were able to take a few successful steps on a walker, and within a week I was able to make it around two-thirds of the rehab gym's perimeter with a normal walker—on my own.

On more than one occasion, I imagined myself back in the ring, except this time, I was fighting a different opponent, one that had nearly taken me out of the game of life altogether.

CHAPTER EIGHTEEN

LIFE LESSONS
FROM WRESTLING

In my younger years I'd always been fascinated by professional wrestling. It was a combination of athleticism and show
business that worked remarkably well together. Growing up
in a small-town (even rural) southern area, there really wasn't
an enormous amount of big-time entertainment. What you
saw at the local theater or on one of the three or four televi-
sion channels you could pick up back then was pretty much it.
Attending professional or even college-level sporting events,
as well as live professional music or performing in any realm,
normally required at least a two-hour drive to a larger city.
There was one notable exception. Professional wrestling.

Back in the sixties, '70s, and well into the '80s, each
section of the country had its own pro wrestling promotion.
The boundaries were established by the outer reaches of the
TV signals of the stations on which they were being broadcast. Each area was governed by whichever promoter operated within these broadcast boundaries. In the Southeast,
this meant Jim Crockett Promotions and Mid-Atlantic

Championship Wrestling. Wrestling aired in the area where I grew up each Saturday afternoon, and everyone who owned a TV set watched it. I wish there would have been a way to do ratings of locally broadcast shows back then. If there had been, I would quickly wager that Saturday afternoon wrestling was right up there at the pinnacle. On Monday morning, you could ask someone how the Yankees or the Braves had done over the weekend, and they may or may not have been able to answer that question correctly. But ask how that tag-team match with Rip Hawk and Swede Hanson against Johnny Weaver and George Becker had ended up, and they sure as hell could respond correctly to that one, thank you. And they'd usually expound quite a bit on all the matches during that one-hour broadcast. They would no doubt go in depth concerning all the dirty tricks and downright dishonest moves used by Hawk and Hanson, and how they just couldn't understand how blind that referee was to not see what was going on right in front of his eyes.

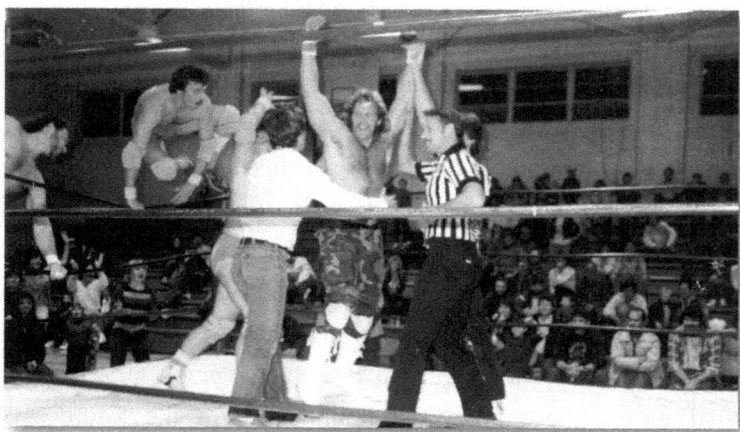

Danny's first pro wrestling match when he won Over the *Top Rope Battle Royal*, Marion, NC, 1986

It was a scenario that played out each week. Good guys get taken advantage of by the bad guys. Sometimes the good guys still came out on top, and sometimes they didn't. Sounds a little like life, huh? It repeated itself Saturday after Saturday and only seemed to increase in popularity. Everybody loved it.

The biggest difference between wrestling and other sports on TV was that matter of a two-hour drive to attend in person. With wrestling this was not the case. Wrestling came right to your hometown high school gym or the closest National Guard Armory. Yep, it came right to your front door. The same guys you saw on the tube the Saturday before would be live—right in your face, beating the hell out of each other. They'd be using (or trying to out-smart) every dirty trick in the book, all for the low, low price of admission, which was usually quite reasonable. It had to be. In the small-town South back then, if they weren't reasonable you just couldn't sell them, and empty seats didn't bring in any money. Promoters like Crockett back then understood this well and made sure you got a quality product for that reasonably priced ticket; and therefore, pro wrestling flourished across the nation.

I, like everyone else, was one of those guys glued to the set each Saturday to watch what the heroes and the dastardly villains were doing. I also got to attend several matches as I was growing up, either at local high schools or in Asheville at the Civic Center. I absolutely loved it! As I look back on it now, I can certainly understand why, because it was the perfect combination of what I enjoyed most: sports and entertainment, both of which were mirrored in my life-path choices.

When Passenger finally came off the road and disbanded in the summer of 1986, I was faced with making some career decisions. I had offers from a couple of other bands and one production company to stay out on the road, mixing live concert sound. I wasn't schooled well enough in the technical aspects of audio engineering to do studio work. However, I'd always adapted well to live sound; so I had no doubt in my mind that I could continue along this path. But I also knew full well that if I chose to do so, things may not turn out so well. Over the previous few years I had witnessed several friends and acquaintances in the music business pass away from varying causes, all related directly to the everyday lifestyle one takes on in that line of work. It was risky unless you were very focused, and I could see I had been losing more focus as time wore on.

I'd moved back in with my parents out of necessity and ended up getting a job in the cotton mill just to be bringing in a paycheck. Humbling, yes, but you did what you had to do. I did have another avenue in mind that I'd always had a great desire to explore, however. Becoming a professional wrestler.

I checked into the best way to get involved in this business, which had always, for subtle reasons, been secretive when it came to its inner operations. Two methods stood out. One, write a fat check to enroll in one of the formal professional wrestling training schools, which were operated across the country by most of the larger promotions; or two, pay a smaller fee and hook up with any of the many small-time operations that dotted the landscape. Like anything else in life, you get what you pay for; and enrolling in the formal school was the obvious way to go . . . but it was much more expensive than I could afford at the time. The nearest school was operated by Crockett Promotions in Mooresville, North Carolina, just north of Charlotte. It cost $200 up front to go through a one-day qualifying tryout; and if you made it through this, it was another $3,300 for the three-month training school.

At any rate, I still wanted to take a shot. I was twenty-seven. I had no wife and, as far as I knew, no kids. No outstanding bills. No major responsibilities of any kind. If I was going to pursue this dream, this would probably be my last chance.

The first thing I had to do was get myself back in excellent physical shape. I had to shake off the effects of nearly five years on the road. I immediately started to work out five days each week at Bracey's gym—the same gym where I'd started serious weight training several years before. These daily workouts, coupled with the physical nature of my job at the mill, brought me along at a pretty rapid pace.

One day I walked into the gym and an old buddy of mine pulled me aside and said, "I've got some info I think you'd be interested in." What he had was the name and a phone number of a local guy who was starting up a small wrestling promotion. I called him and he said for $100 they'd train me in the basics and get me some exposure when they thought I was ready. I couldn't turn it down. I started my training that same week.

The training was more physical than I had expected. Learning how to repeatedly throw your body onto a solid surface without being injured is actually quite difficult. Your mind is telling your body that it's not supposed to fall and therefore your body wants to cooperate because it has no reason to disbelieve a mind that's always made sound safety decisions in the past. It was difficult, but I eventually got my mind and body to come into agreement.

I progressed rapidly in my role as a "babyface." That's wrestling lingo for a good guy. A bad guy is referred to as a "heel." At first, I didn't even know that much. I told you, pro wrestling was very secretive, and there were good reasons for it. Most of the folks buying tickets believed everything they were watching was absolutely genuine. We were taught that the word *fake* was not in our vocabulary and we would not tolerate this blasphemous term used in our presence. This is one reason I no longer watch wrestling. Now it's nothing more than a long string of interviews interlaced with over-the-top visual and audio production, and a few incredible acrobatic moves thrown in for good measure. There's no storyline whatsoever; and worst of all, they even admit it's all fake. In my mind, this is completely out the question.

As I progressed, I started to get a fair amount of publicity; and before long I was able to quit the old day job and turn to wrestling as a full-time gig. In an effort to improve my product even more, I was accepted into Crockett's training school after passing the one-day qualifying event.

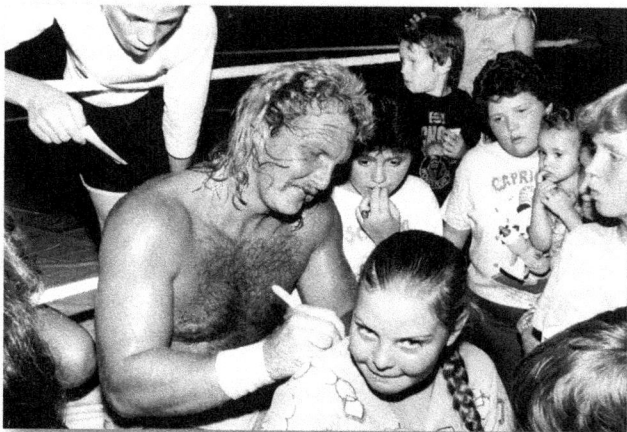

Danny signing autographs for adoring fans, 1987

Let me make one thing perfectly clear. The bodily torture they put me through that day was without a doubt the most difficult physical event of my life. I only *thought* I was in shape. It was pure hell. I found out later that they could have made it even more difficult on me. But they liked my look and the fact that I had already learned the basics and performed in front of a crowd on many occasions. On the outside, this qualifying event may just seem like a way to make a quick $200, as most quit the first day. It's actually a requirement. Your finished product must justify the ticket price paid by the fan who wants to see you pushed to the limit every time you step into the ring. In order to produce a quality product each and every night, quitting is not an option.

Overall, wrestling was an enjoyable experience, and I stayed in it for about two and a half years. I would have hung in there longer except for a couple of reasons. The money wasn't nearly as big back then as it turned out to be after the advent of cable TV, which transformed it into a national and even worldwide event. The other reason may sound a little strange, but I'll attempt to explain. Wrestling was a boring lifestyle. I was constantly on the road, much as had been the case with music. That was nothing new as I had stayed with music for several years. So what was the difference when it came to wrestling? In music you're on stage or directly involved in a show that goes on for hours and often in the same town for multiple days. In wrestling, you're in the ring for generally less than a half hour. The rest of the time you're either in a dressing room, a hotel, or a car; and it was always a series of one-nighters. I'd had enough of living out of a suitcase, so I decided to hang it up.

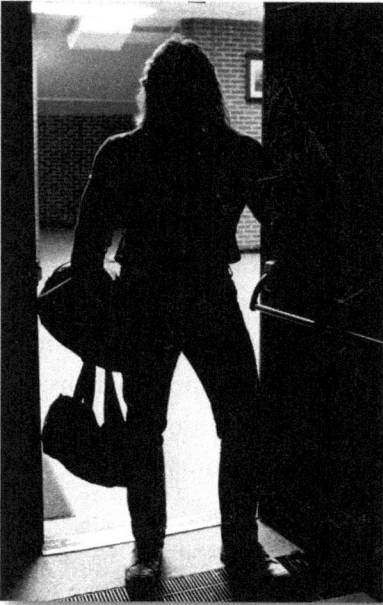

Danny leaving the arena (photo by late Steve Dixon).
Asheville, NC, 1986

One thing will forever be etched in my mind in regard to professional wrestling—one thing I witnessed that nothing will ever erase. It created a feeling in my body and soul that will probably never be duplicated, and it involves that blasphemous term I spoke of earlier. *Fake.*

I was sixteen years old and had taken my youngest brother to the Civic Center in Asheville to watch that week's card. The main event was the babyface, "Chief" Wahoo McDaniel facing the heel, Greg "The Hammer" Valentine. Wahoo was the classic good guy, especially in Asheville due to its proximity to the Cherokee Indian Reservation; and the bad guys didn't get any dastardlier or more vicious than Valentine. These guys were masters of their craft. Chief Wahoo walked into the arena to a booming ovation in front of a sold out crowd of 8000. The place was going nuts. He danced around inside the ring with his full headdress, much to the delight of everyone in the building. After a short wait came Valentine slowly strutting in, wearing a full-length velvet robe with "The Hammer" boldly embroidered across the back. Valentine took his time walking up to the steps that led up to the ring, flipping his long bleach-blond hair around like a super model on a runway. The boos raining down on him were deafening. He slowly placed his right foot on the first step and his right hand on the bottom ring rope, stopped dead cold and locked eyes with Wahoo, who stood perfectly motionless in the center of the ring with his hands on his hips. The noise from the crowd suddenly dissipated to absolute silence. You could have heard a pin drop. The tension was so thick you could have cut it with a knife. After a few seconds, Valentine slowly began his next step . . . and the noise inside the Civic Center slowly swelled to thunderous proportions—and at that moment, my friends, professional wrestling was real indeed.

***

Unfortunately, around the time I began walking in rehab, I also got a visit from my caseworker informing me that I had progressed to the point that Blue Cross would no longer pay for continued in-house therapy. I would be discharged on March 4th.

I was actually disappointed that I'd be leaving, as I was making so much progress and was truly enjoying everybody's company; but going back home after six months was an appealing thought. So, I went around and told everyone how much I loved them, thanking them for everything they'd done for me. I knew I'd miss them, but all good things must come to an end.

The night before I was discharged it started to snow in Asheville, and as I sat there in my manual wheelchair (yes, I had moved up in this area too), I had a lot of time to reflect. Just six months before I'd been hit with some out-of-the-blue illness that I'd never even heard of, and I had nearly died in the process. I'd lost all my physical abilities, both voluntary and involuntary. I had been all over the country and part way around the world during my most varied life, but I suddenly found myself in a place I'd never envisioned whatsoever. But I was still alive; and with the help of those around me, I was able to leave this difficult season behind. Many people ask me what I learned from my experience, and what I can honestly convey to you is this: do not take life for granted. It can be taken away in a flash. Get everything you can out of life today because there may be no tomorrow. But in doing so, treat others as you want to be treated. Let the actions of others determine how you perceive them, but don't form opinions before you get to know them. In other words, just try to live as good a life as you can—and don't ever lose faith in yourself. We all have a lot more down deep inside us than we think we do. When you go to bed at the end of the day, if you've lived that day in this manner, then you can fall off to sleep knowing you've accomplished your goal for that day. When it all comes down to it, that's about all any of us can do. I went to bed that night feeling pretty good about things.

The next morning, to my surprise, I wasn't awoken by the first-shift nurses but rather by pool friends Reta, Lee, and Megan. They'd come to tell me goodbye, wish me luck, and tell me how much they had enjoyed meeting me and working with me. I think I shed a couple of tears—and wasn't embarrassed at all to do so. Several others stopped by to bid me good luck as well, and I was appreciative of each and every one. I got out of bed and into my wheelchair, realizing that for the first time in two months there was no daily schedule taped to it. I guess it was time to start making my own schedules again.

Duane arrived to pick me up about 10:30, and Leslie walked down to the car with me in my wheelchair to say goodbye. No, I hadn't accomplished my goal of walking out the front door on my own. Can't win 'em all. But I sure as hell gave it my best. All my stuff was loaded and I transferred over into the passenger's seat of my own car. Duane had driven it up that day, and this was the first time I wouldn't be the pilot in my own car on my way home. I was a passenger for the first time. It felt a little strange, but those days a lot of things felt strange.

Once we were on I-40 headed home, Duane told me to reach behind his seat and see what was back there. I found a small cooler containing two cold Michelob Ultras, my beer of choice at the time. I promptly thanked him and popped the top on what would be the first beer I'd tasted in a half year. Man, it tasted good! Frothy, refreshing, totally satisfying. Then it hit me. You know, no matter how good that beer tasted, it didn't—and never will—quite top that Coke on ice just a couple of months before.

EPILOGUE

I still remember the first time I got on a roller coaster. I was a teenager at an amusement park called Carowinds, located just below Charlotte, North Carolina. The name of the ride was Thunder Road. It was one of the old roller coasters made of wood, the park's flagship attraction for many years. It's been torn down; but the memory of my first time on it can never be torn away from my mind, just as the events that occurred during my battle with and rehabilitation from Guillain-Barré Syndrome will always be cemented into my memory.

As I look back on it all today, taking a ride on a roller coaster and how I've lived my life resemble each other—and very much so. You get that bar locked across your lap once you're in the car; and it starts to inch forward slowly, picking up speed—just as your thoughts are starting to accelerate as well. Then you finally come to that first long climb to an apex that disappears into the sky above. The sound of the chain clicking along as it pulls those cars up that incline is a sound that cannot be mistaken for any other. It is unique. The anticipation builds for what's ahead, and once you've come to a near stop at the top . . . suddenly the bottom drops out and you find yourself helplessly hurtling back toward the same earth that it seemed you were just leaving a second before.

Your heart comes up into your throat and you're faced with the realization that if the least thing goes awry—this could be the end of the story.

However, in an instant you bottom out and are slung into a hairpin turn, which throws you against the side of the car—or the side of your companion in the car, should you have one. This is followed by several more peaks and valleys and sharp turns until finally the finish point is in sight. You finally experience a feeling of welcome safety but at the same time a desire comes from way down inside your gut to get back in line and ride it again! Do you get back on or not? You've finished something that very well could have killed you! You could have bought the farm! Do you get back on or not?

As I have sought to describe in my writings, the choices I made in my life and the things I experienced were, for the most part, certainly not ordinary. But they may have, in a quite unintentional manner, prepared me for the greatest challenge I'd ever confront.

In 1986 I attended the ten-year reunion of my high school graduating class. Nearly all my class-mates had taken the con-ventional road of getting married and starting a family. Most seemed

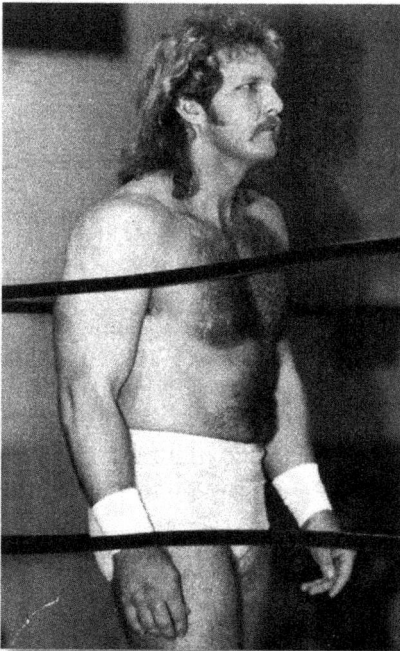

Danny as a professional wrestler, 1987

happy but appeared to be a little bored as well. I, on the other hand, was anything but bored. I was twenty-seven and had already been the top assistant manager of a 35,000-square-foot department store, a long-haul truck driver, a bouncer/bartender, and—for the previous five years—the road manager and sound engineer of a traveling rock band. I was about to become a professional wrestler. I had no family, and I had no solid career in place; but I certainly wasn't bored.

As time continued, my life did take on some semblance of normalcy and finally stabilized once I began my employment with the Department of Correction. The roller coaster ride leveled out at that point and it looked as if I would just slowly roll under the shaded, roofed-over area that housed the finish line.

On September 24, 2015, I found myself locked into that coaster car, hurtling out of control toward a ground I was unable to make out—and I hadn't even heard the clicking of the chain pulling me upward. I never saw it coming. But I didn't give up.

As I write this, it's been four years since that fateful day in 2015. I've come a long way; and I'm now self-sufficient, even though I'm still not quite as good as new. I've had my share of setbacks and still live with a considerable amount of pain and decreased mobility. But I do, in fact, still live. Actually, I'm able to maintain a satisfying and somewhat active life. I go to our local YMCA five times a week, where I normally spend two to three hours. I do my fair share of socializing, but—make no mistake about it—I get my money's worth too, as evidenced by the sweat-soaked T-shirt on my back as I leave each day.

I feel that I still maintain a productive life as well. I may never be able to work a job that requires a certain amount of manual labor again, but who knows? Maybe I will. I seem to be progressing a little more most days and I like to attempt something new just to see if I can pull it off. Sometimes I can and sometimes I can't, but at least I can still make the attempt. Being involved in a productive lifestyle is very important to me (I wrote this book, didn't I?), and I wish it were important to more people. The world would be better off. Nothing bad can come from drive, determination, and effort.

I thank you for reading of my experience, and I hope you have not only enjoyed what you've read, but perhaps even gained a bit of inspiration and insight from it.

Now back to my earlier question. Would I get back on that roller coaster, or would I perhaps choose a smoother, calmer ride? Would I get back on?

IN A HEARTBEAT!

ACKNOWLEDGEMENTS

I would like to thank each of you for reading my story.

Thanks to the doctors, nurses, therapists, and all the professionals who assisted me through this odyssey. You did not give up on me. You will always be remembered, and I hope you will remember me.

Thanks also to all of you who were instrumental in my upbringing and life experiences. First of all, my parents, and also my friends, co-workers, teammates, and others who have helped to shape who I am today.

ABOUT THE AUTHOR

Danny Freeman lives in his childhood home in Nebo, North Carolina. He typed this entire manuscript with his two index fingers from a wheelchair at his desk. He doesn't need the wheelchair anymore, but he says it's the most comfortable seat to type in. He still loves music, sports, travel, and the company of women—who, as evidenced by several lifelong friendships, attest to the fact that they still love him too. He can size you up within seconds of your first conversation; and if he trusts you, you'll be the recipient of more genuine companionship and life stories than we could fit into this book, accompanied by his contagious laughter and positive outlook on life.

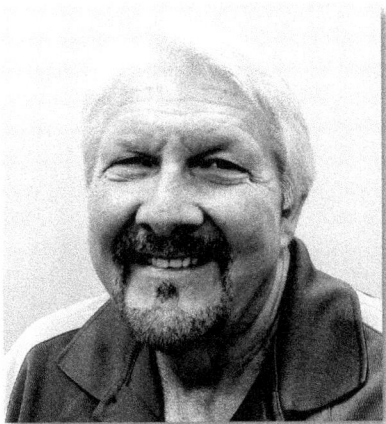